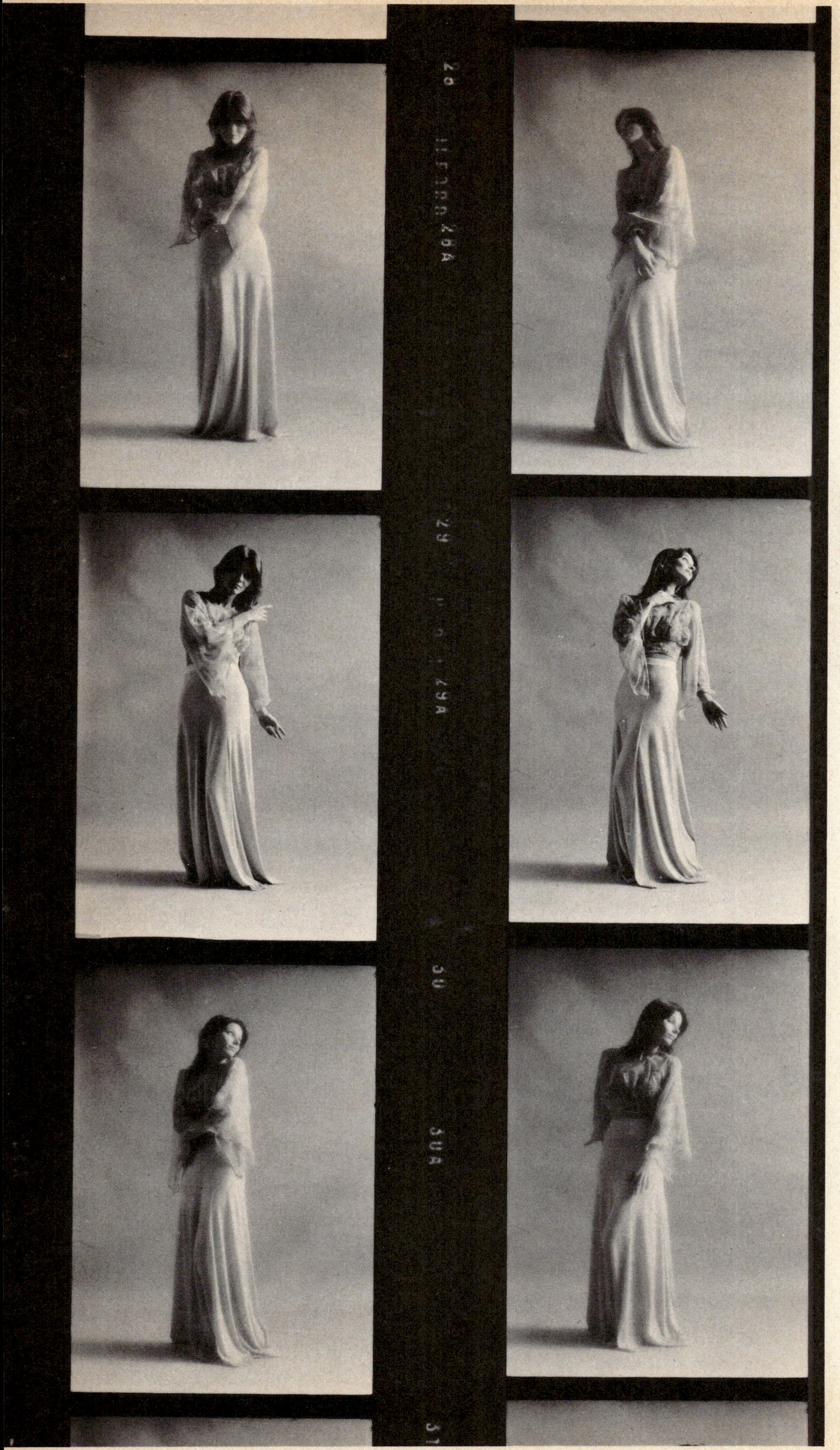

photographic
modeling
by
valerie
cragin

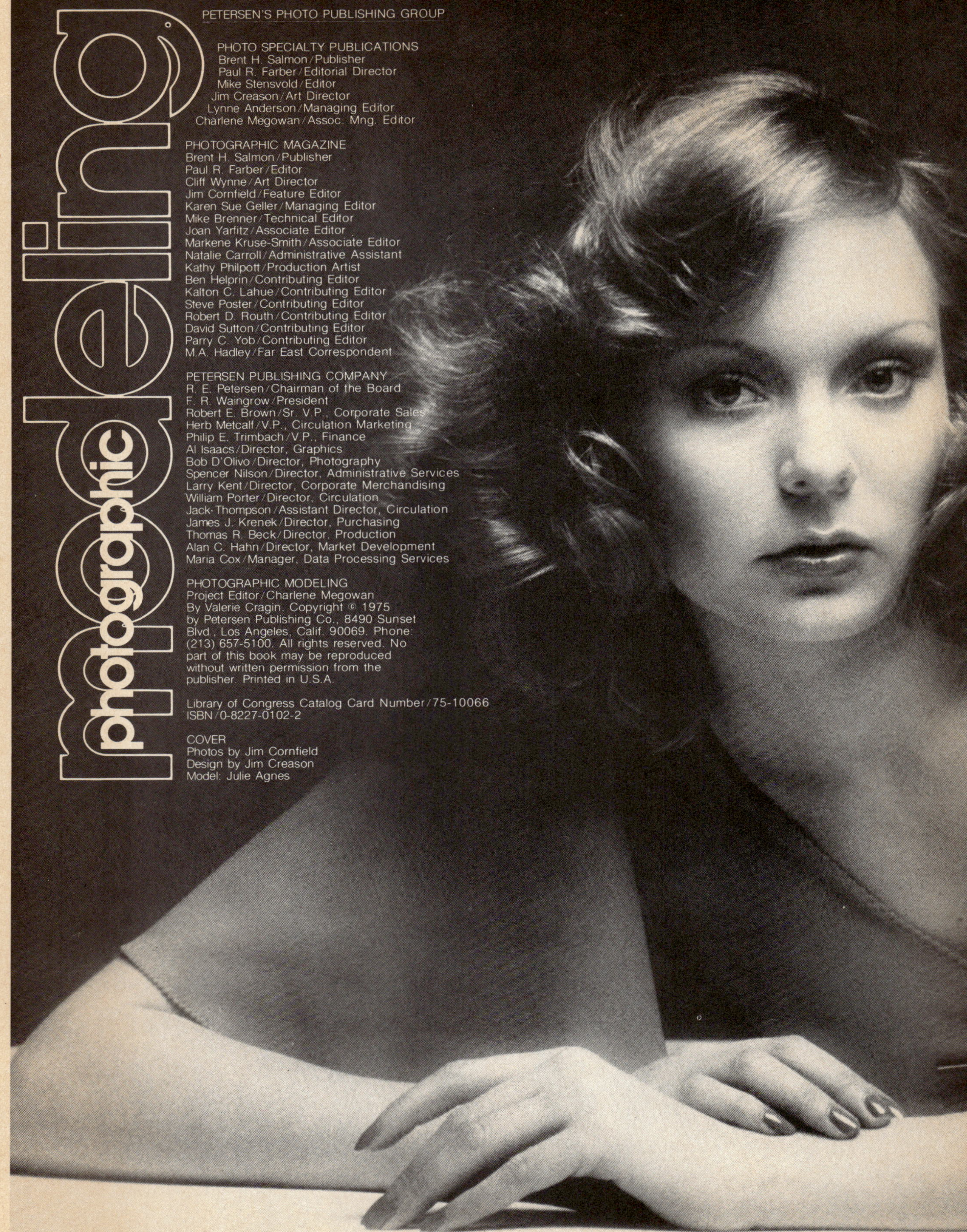

photographic modeling

PETERSEN'S PHOTO PUBLISHING GROUP

PHOTO SPECIALTY PUBLICATIONS
Brent H. Salmon/Publisher
Paul R. Farber/Editorial Director
Mike Stensvold/Editor
Jim Creason/Art Director
Lynne Anderson/Managing Editor
Charlene Megowan/Assoc. Mng. Editor

PHOTOGRAPHIC MAGAZINE
Brent H. Salmon/Publisher
Paul R. Farber/Editor
Cliff Wynne/Art Director
Jim Cornfield/Feature Editor
Karen Sue Geller/Managing Editor
Mike Brenner/Technical Editor
Joan Yarfitz/Associate Editor
Markene Kruse-Smith/Associate Editor
Natalie Carroll/Administrative Assistant
Kathy Philpott/Production Artist
Ben Helprin/Contributing Editor
Kalton C. Lahue/Contributing Editor
Steve Poster/Contributing Editor
Robert D. Routh/Contributing Editor
David Sutton/Contributing Editor
Parry C. Yob/Contributing Editor
M.A. Hadley/Far East Correspondent

PETERSEN PUBLISHING COMPANY
R. E. Petersen/Chairman of the Board
F. R. Waingrow/President
Robert E. Brown/Sr. V.P., Corporate Sales
Herb Metcalf/V.P., Circulation Marketing
Philip E. Trimbach/V.P., Finance
Al Isaacs/Director, Graphics
Bob D'Olivo/Director, Photography
Spencer Nilson/Director, Administrative Services
Larry Kent/Director, Corporate Merchandising
William Porter/Director, Circulation
Jack Thompson/Assistant Director, Circulation
James J. Krenek/Director, Purchasing
Thomas R. Beck/Director, Production
Alan C. Hahn/Director, Market Development
Maria Cox/Manager, Data Processing Services

PHOTOGRAPHIC MODELING
Project Editor/Charlene Megowan
By Valerie Cragin. Copyright © 1975
by Petersen Publishing Co., 8490 Sunset
Blvd., Los Angeles, Calif. 90069. Phone:
(213) 657-5100. All rights reserved. No
part of this book may be reproduced
without written permission from the
publisher. Printed in U.S.A.

Library of Congress Catalog Card Number/75-10066
ISBN/0-8227-0102-2

COVER
Photos by Jim Cornfield
Design by Jim Creason
Model: Julie Agnes

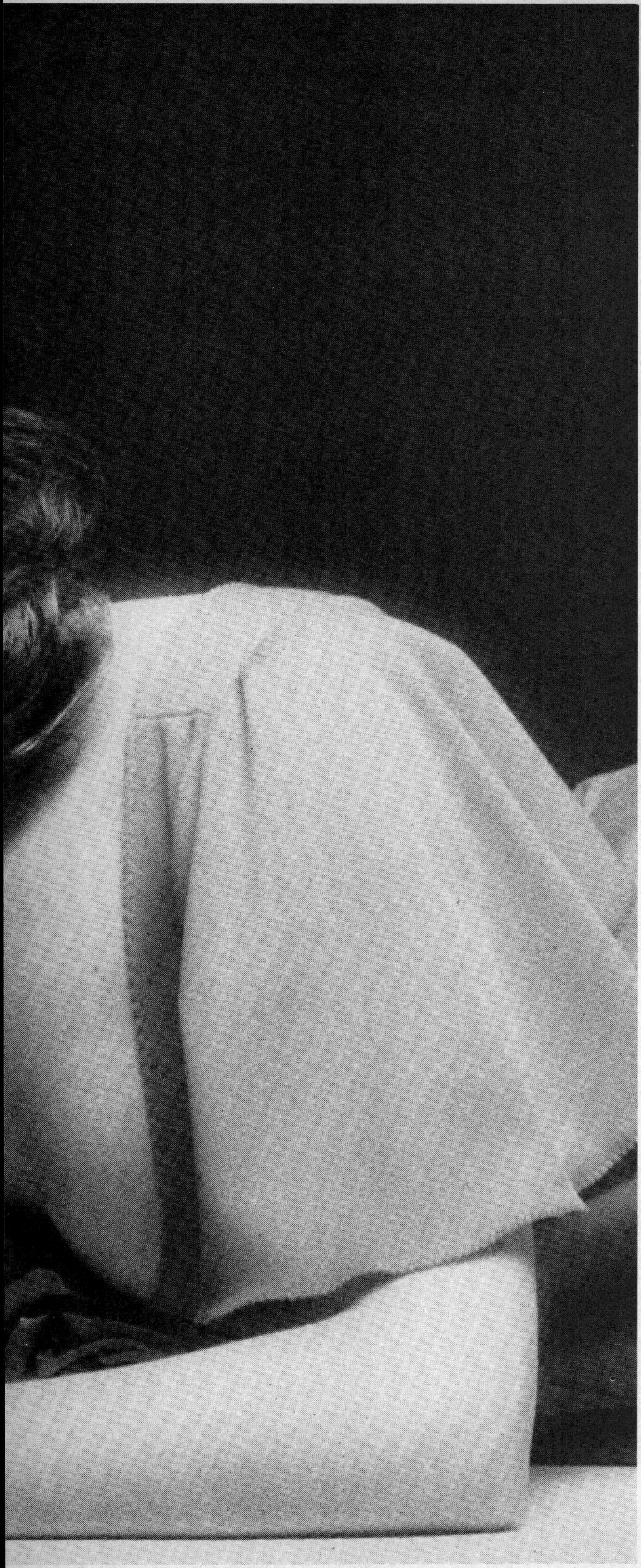

introduction

The photographic artist presents his perception of life and beauty around him. He captures, within a small frame, a moment of life or a segment of nature or architecture that particularly intrigues him and personalizes the content within the frame by his selection of photographic angles, lighting, focus and perhaps color.

These pages are devoted to the photographer who would like to develop style and perfect techniques in working with a model as an element of a picture (as in a situational shot, scenic study, fashion or magazine layout) in which the model is either integral or of

Properly used, the model will become the center of communication between the photographer and the viewer.

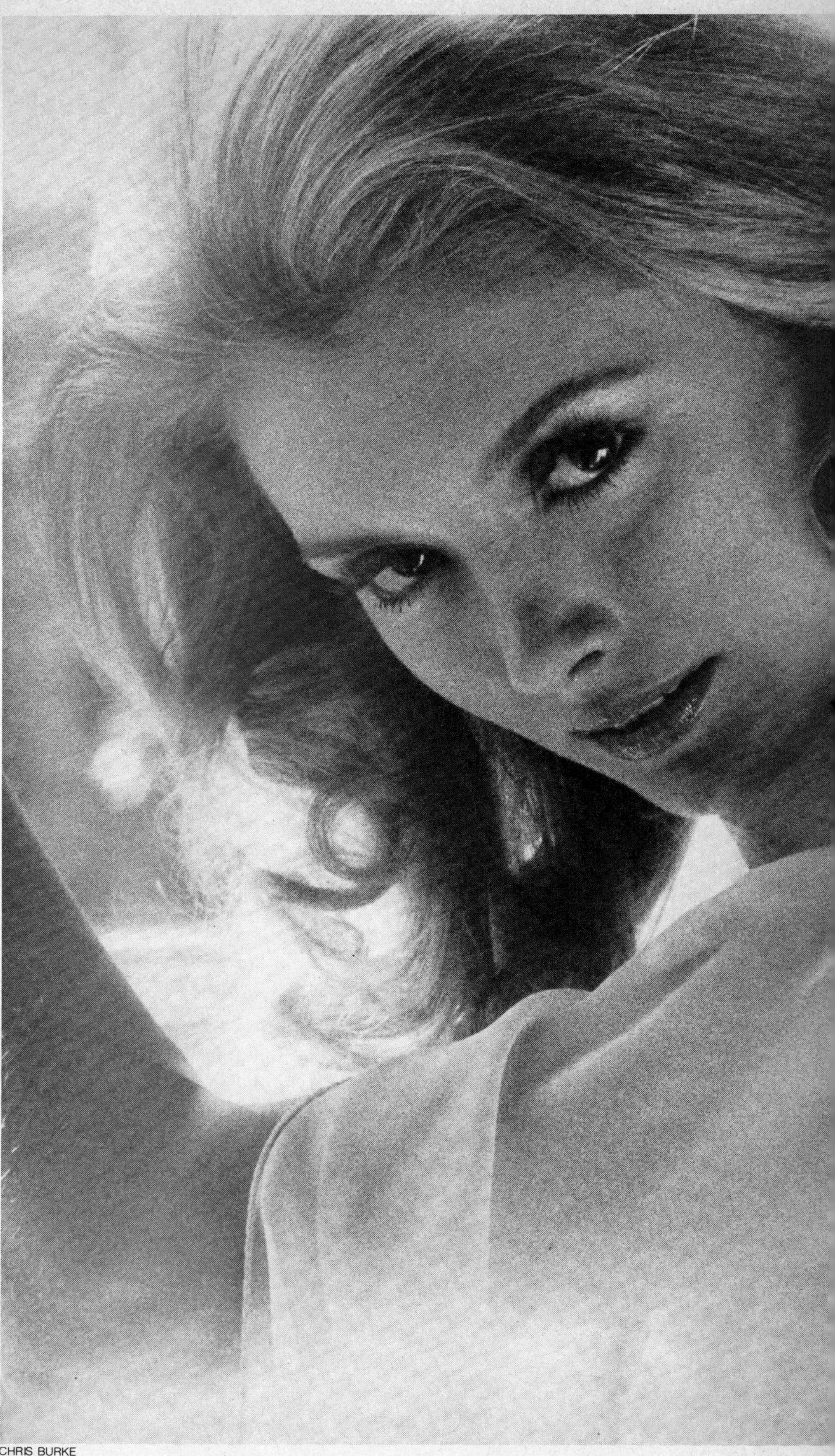
CHRIS BURKE

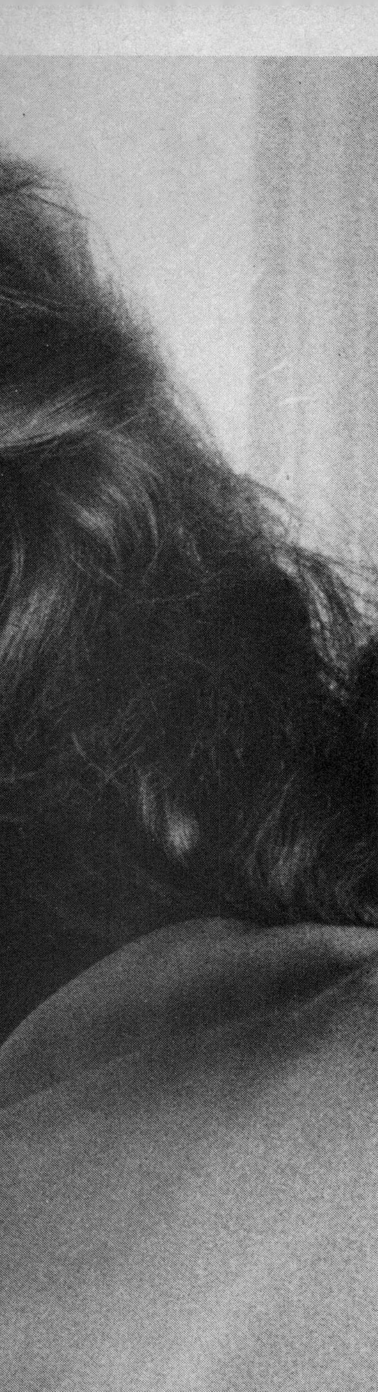

incidental interest to the picture—rather than the sole interest of the picture, as in portraiture.

A photographic model not only brings life to a photograph, but, correctly chosen and directed, can also lend color, mood, symmetry of line, fluidity of suspended movement, and express a relationship to the selected environment. In addition, the viewer tends to relate to the model in recalling an event or mood, thus making the model the center of communication between the photographer and the viewer.

The photographer who has access to expensive, fully trained, experienced professional models has obvious advantages. But every model has to be trained and developed at the early stages of her career and, mostly, it's the photographer who is working with the novice model who makes the most meaningful contribution to her development.

This book is addressed to the photographer who would like to help the models he works with to become more effective and of professional caliber in physical appearance, ability to create moods and body movements. And finally, to the models who understand that great pictures are the result of the perfectly balanced, mutual creative efforts of both the photographer and the model. □

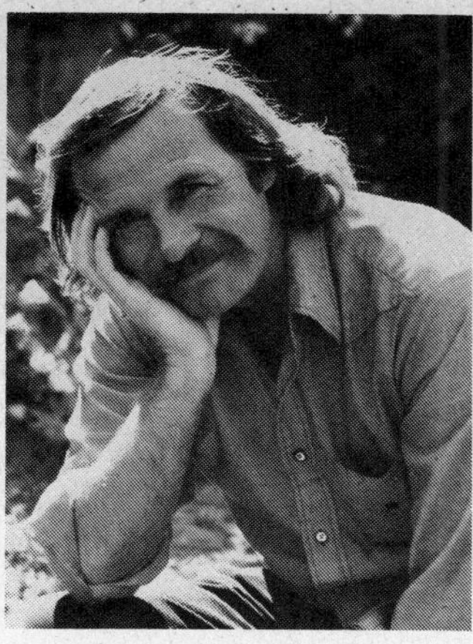

The Photographer: Ed Johannes, who shot the pictures in this book, is particularly well equipped to understand photographers' problems with novice models. As director of photography for the Flaire Modeling Agency for the past nine years, he has patiently counseled and directed literally thousands of fledgling models in their first in-front-of-camera experiences. In addition, Ed has many commercial accounts.

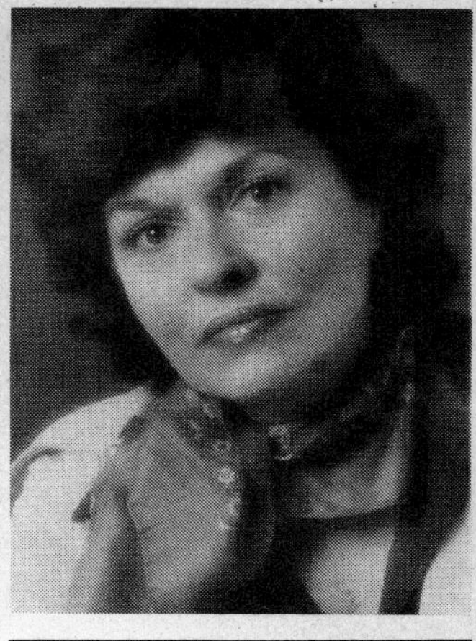

The Author: Valerie Cragin, president of the Flaire Modeling School, Inc. and the Flaire Agency, has trained and represented more than 12,000 girls in the modeling field in the past 20 years.

Formerly a successful model herself, she understands the problems of the model as well as the photographer and stylist.

Valerie is a distinguished lecturer and authority on beauty, fashion and charm, and has written articles for PhotoGraphic and Teen magazines and the Los Angeles Times. In addition, she has written books on charm and modeling for several department stores, and produced the fashion segment of the Noon News with Jack Latham on KTTV for several years.

the importance of rapport

It is of utmost importance that a photographer and the model or models he is working with establish a mutual understanding and appreciation of each other. This good rapport not only makes the time spent on the project enjoyable, but the artistic effect will benefit considerably.

The photographer and the model should consider the mood of the project, and try to establish an atmosphere in accordance with it.

When the assignment is to be romantic, poetic, soft shots, the photographer can help his model by acting in the gentlest, most courtly manner possible. Arrange to have some soft music playing, keep the voices soft, joking down to a minimum. Recognize her needs as an actress and your own needs as an artist in capturing the expression of a special quality and mood.

The general tone of an outdoor, sporty assignment, on the other hand, should inspire a feeling of freedom, fun, vigor and well-being. Kid with her, convince her you appreciate her humor—while still appealing to her vanity as a beautiful person. (If she starts to clown around too much, a lot of film might be wasted on funny faces.)

It's important that the kidding around doesn't take on a too-fresh tone on the part of the photographer. (It may seem that she is amused; but there is a very real risk that she's concealing embarrassment, resentment, or is becoming defensive.) If photographers could only eavesdrop on a group of models comparing notes about which photographers are too *grabby* and which ones think they're every model's special sexual fantasy, they would possibly exercise a little

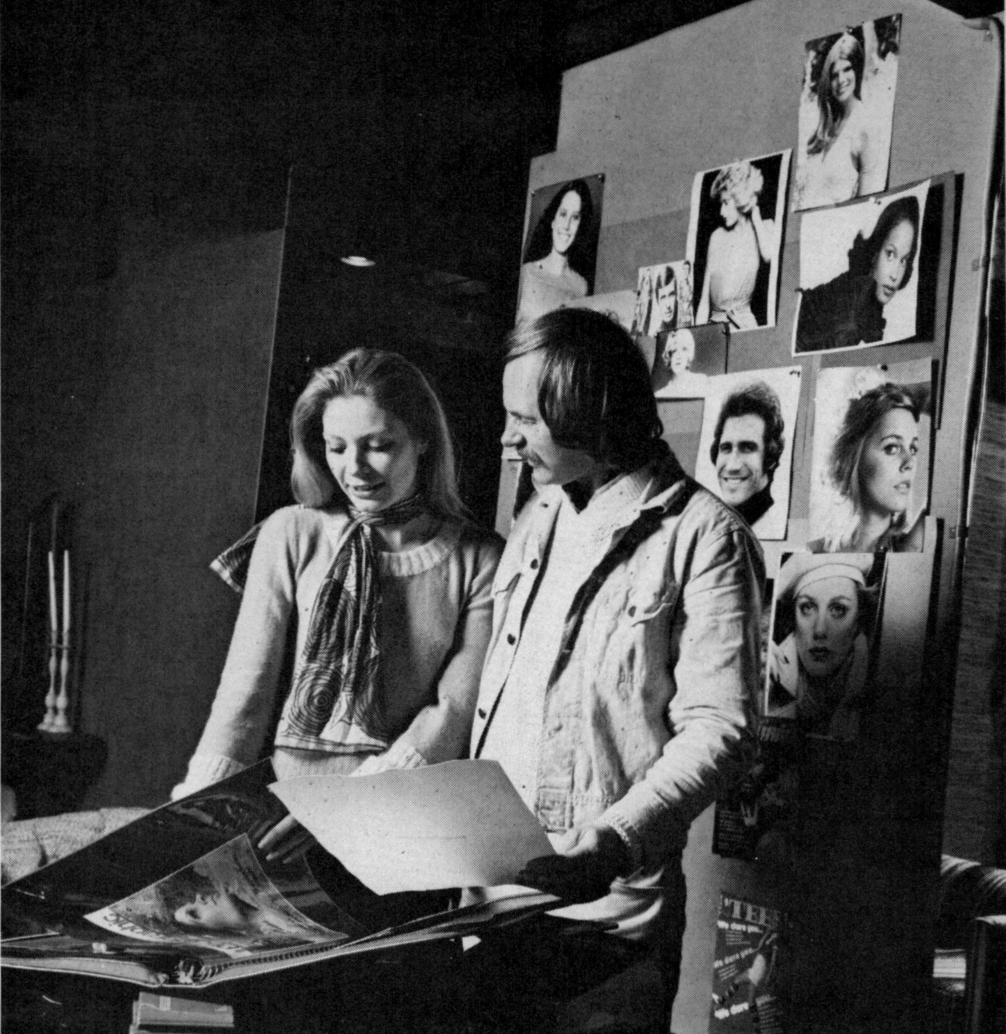

JON MARLOW AND ED JOHANNES

more sensitivity in this area. It's undeniably advantageous when a female model and a male photographer experience a mutual attraction for each other—but it is most effective when its an unexpressed undercurrent—and she feels totally safe in flirting with the man behind the camera.

Along with the very personal relationship between the photographer and model, there must also be a strong professional respect. Professional courtesy and consideration are maintained before, during and after the shooting.

A comfortable dressing area should be provided, and the photographer should respect the privacy of the model. (No crashing in on her while she's dressing with, "It's okay, honey, I'm just like your doctor," or, "I see it all the time.") Most models resent it.

Consideration of the model's comfort should always be shown—especially during outdoor shooting. Bring a towel and warm robe

if you're going to ask her to freeze in the ocean at dawn—let her rest between shots if she's tired—have a Thermos of lemonade or ice water for hot days and coffee or hot chocolate for cold—arrange to have sandwiches with you if your location might not have a restaurant nearby. Cranky, hungry models don't photograph well. Be kind, thoughtful and businesslike, and good dividends will appear in your photos.

Models, on the other hand, have definite attitudinal responsibilities toward the photographer and the

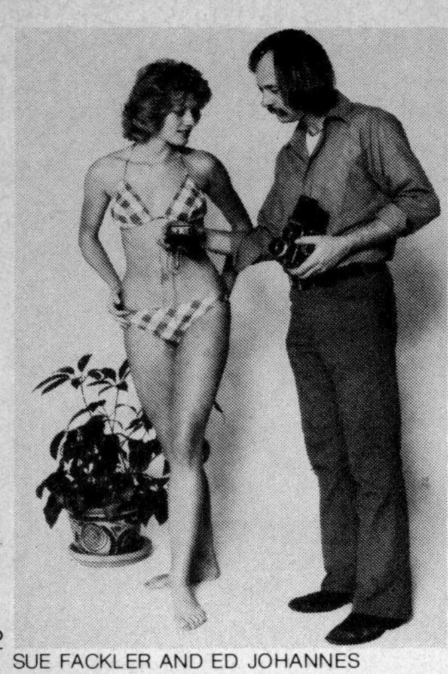

2

SUE FACKLER AND ED JOHANNES

1. Interviewing the model should be done in a businesslike but relaxed atmosphere, preferably in a studio or office.
2. Good rapport between photographer and model makes the time spent on a project enjoyable and the artistic effect will benefit considerably as well.

assignment. The model must arrive on time, completely prepared, and with enthusiasm and eagerness toward the assignment.

She must convey an impression of confidence, a sincere desire to please, and a willingness to happily make every effort possible to ensure success to the project.

Sometimes, photographic modeling (especially on location) can entail minor physical discomfort—i.e., working under hot lights in a fur coat, nearly freezing on a beach or in the water on a clear but cold day or dancing around in sticky weeds with bare feet, etc. A model must be a good sport throughout it all. Any unwillingness to cooperate on her part is sensed both by the photographer and his camera, and can ruin the shot. Of course, too, there must be enough honesty and trust between the photographer and model for her to feel free to tell him if the request seems unreasonable.

A special warning to photographers using a loved one as a model—this particular situation is loaded with trouble, and handled improperly, can result in lost shots as well as endangered relationships. In this case,

your model is in the most vulnerable of all situations. She must now expose the fantasy side of her nature to the man who has already approved of the real girl. She's risking her lover as well as her pride. Take it *very* easy with criticism— encourage her, flatter her, let her know you now love her more than ever after viewing her through the camera. It will pay dividends in good pictures as well as those of a more personal nature.

INTERVIEWING THE MODEL

Modeling interviews can be painful experiences for both the photographer and the models. However, when each of them approaches the initial interview with the determination to make it a pleasant encounter for the other person, it can be a delightful experience.

The photographer should provide a businesslike, but relaxed atmosphere for the initial interview. Understandably, most models are a bit apprehensive about meeting with a strange photographer in his home, at a restaurant, or in a hotel room. Very attractive girls, both inside and outside of the modeling profession, soon learn to avoid compromising situations—and, although your intentions might be totally honorable, the model generally prefers not to make a social occasion of an interview.

If the photographer does not have a real studio, he might try to borrow one, use the client's (if there is one) or a friend's office, the

building used by the camera club for meetings or the room where your camera classes are held. If she is a professional model represented by an agent, the agency is usually happy to make arrangements for the two of you to meet at the agency office.

The photographer should remember that the model might very likely be nervous and apprehensive. After all, she's placing herself in the very vulnerable position of being accepted or rejected.

The photographer should always try to convey the impression that he approves of some aspect of the model; albeit she may not be his choice for that particular project.

The professional model (and even many semipros) will bring her portfolio for the photographer's inspection. Many photographers make the terrible mistake of criticizing the pictures in the portfolio. It is tactless, inconsiderate, and totally devoid of understanding that this is simply the best she has to offer. If the pictures are really poor and the photographer is prepared to test the model himself and give her some prints, he can tell her that she's beautiful, but he doesn't think any photographer has done her justice. There are right and wrong ways to say things:

SHE'S OVERWEIGHT—Don't tell her she's fat! *Do* tell her she has a lovely figure but, the camera adds weight to a girl so your particular needs this time are for a slimmer model and you would love to see her again when and if she loses 10 to 15 pounds.

HER HAIR IS A TERRIBLE COLOR—Don't tell her it's overbleached or dyed. *Do* tell her that her face is so lovely that, in your opinion, her features would be set off by a softer shade of hair color.

SHE DOESN'T HAVE ENOUGH EXPERIENCE— Don't make her feel like a rank amateur. *Do* let her know you think she's terrific,

but this project is going to require some very fast, hectic shooting and this time you will have to limit yourself to using an experienced girl—and you want to save her for an assignment when you can spend some real time working with her.

Of course, the very simplest answer to all of these and any other reasons for rejection is: ''Thank you for coming in; we have to see some other models; but we do think you're lovely and will call your agency (or will call you, if she's not represented) if we can use you.''

An agency representing a model takes the heat off the photographer—if he has any constructive criticism, the smart agent will appreciate the comments. If the model or the agent is not receptive to your suggestions, don't force it. After all, it's just one photographer's opinion. Other photographers might possibly have said the opposite.

Although tact is always in order, flattery frequently desirable, deceit is unforgivable. Don't be a coward and make false promises to the model.

Repeated experiences of broken promises tend to make the model lose confidence in herself and she needs as much self-esteem as she can possibly muster to pursue a successful career.

Also, it's possible that you may decide to use her after all in the future, and it would be unfortunate if she had learned to mistrust you.

If the model interviewed is a novice, she most likely will not have a portfolio to show you or a composite to leave with you so you can remember her. In this instance, if you are at all interested, we highly recommend taking at least a Polaroid shot of her for your records.

The best conversational opener is the photographer's current project itself. Describe to the girl the kind of photographs you're planning. Try to determine her reactions to your ideas. Before, during, and after the conversation let her feel that you approve of her. Find a nice feature and compliment her. It's best to stay away from subjects that are too personal at first. "Are you married, do you live with your folks or a roommate, how old are you, are you going steady with someone?"—all may very well be questions you truly want to ask. Ask later. Right at first, the professional relationship might suffer if she feels you're more interested in finding a girl friend than a model. That's flying under false colors and using a ruse. Most every girl resents it. Later on, your professional friendship might very well become a personal friendship. But, at that stage of your relationship, the girl is going to know that the personal friendship is based on mutual respect—not trickery or opportunism.

From time to time, a professional photographer is required to interview many models for a particular assignment. In the trade, these are known (bitterly) as "cattle-calls." And, indeed, some photographers do herd the models through the interview as if they were cattle on the way to the slaughterhouse instead of sensitive, dignified, respectable people. Whenever possible,

arrangements should be made for the models to be interviewed at least 10 minutes apart. An assistant should be on hand to help sign in the models at the time of arrival and check the times of their appointments. On all interviews, it's desirable to have the model fill out an application stating name, phone where she can be reached*, height, size, measurements, coloring and special abilities in sports or the dance.

*If the model is represented by an agency, it is frequently considered bad professional technique to request her home telephone number and address. The name of her agent and the agent's phone number is all that should be required.

GIVING DIRECTIONS

PRIOR TO SHOOTING—A large part of the success of a photographic project is determined by the photographer's ability to communicate to the model specific directions which she can easily understand. Prior to the shooting session, all arrangements must be clarified and confirmed. The model must be told the exact time she should report to the studio or location, where to report (if it's a location, specific directions must be given), what she should bring with her, the nature of the project, makeup and hair requirements, how long the shooting is expected to take, whether or not the project is on a weather-permitting basis and whom to contact if there is any question about the weather. The model's fees (whether she is to receive actual monetary consideration or simply prints) should be firmly

established—with the agency, if she is represented (including billing information), or with the individual model, if she has no representation. (In that case, it should be preestablished as to who will pay her and when.)

Full and absolute communication ahead of time will assure a good start to the shooting. A confusing beginning often affects the entire project's success.

ON THE SCENE—The model should never get in front of the camera until she fully understands what the photographer has in mind. Occasionally, an artistic rendering of a layout is presented by an advertising agency and the model and photographer should look it over carefully so they can present an exact photographic rendition of the artists' concept along with some variations on the theme that will provide some choice to the client.

More often, however, the concept of the shot is only in the photographer's mind. He should try to visualize the shot in his imagination and describe it as clearly as possible to the model. Once working, they might mutually decide to depart from the exacting requirements of the photographer's original concept and express some spontaneous inspirations in movement and mood. The photographer and model should both be open to *things that just happen* during a shooting. Depending upon the rapport and artistic potential of the shot, the photographer and model might find themselves expressing a seemingly limitless number of original and spontaneous ideas.

The photographer should allow the model to express herself as fully as she is capable of doing within the framework of the desired result. But even the finest of models needs the help of the photographer's eye and viewpoint to refine her poses. When giving

directions, the photographer should be patient and concise. Remembering that their positions are reversed, he should refer clearly to the right or left arm or leg.

The photographer can teach the less experienced model to make very gradual corrections by telling her the degree of movement he desires. In other words, not, "Bring your left arm down," or, "Lower your left arm," but, "Bring your left arm down very slowly—just a little bit, until I tell you to stop—okay, stop."

Sometimes, it helps the model to retain her confidence if the photographer has time to explain why he needs an alteration in her position such as, "Let's move your head a little to the left—there's a sunspot on your face," or, "I'll catch a beautiful shadow if you lean just a bit further back."

Make the directions loud and clear if you don't want your model to ruin a pose by leaning forward to ask, "What did you say?" When an alteration of a garment is required, the photographer should make it clear whether he wants the model to correct the problem or if he wants her to stay in place so the photographer (or preferably, the stylist if there is one) can make the adjustment.

Some models (especially inexperienced ones) are a little touchy about the photographer making adjustments to clothing, especially if the necessary adjustment is around the bustline, waist, or hips. It's tactful for the photographer to state what is wrong prior to touching her and ask if she minds.

THE NUDE MODEL

Ideally, a photographer should work with a model several times, fully clad, prior to asking her to work in the nude. This procedure gives the photographer the chance to establish a feeling of mutual trust. He has the opportunity to establish the fact that he respects her, admires her, and a professional rapport is developed. When the subject of nude modeling is broached, it's best if the photographer has a specific project in mind and can clearly describe it to the model so she will feel certain that the results of the shooting are going to be in good taste and her nudity has some artistic justification.

Either the model is or is not willing to do nudes—and, if she is at all reluctant, she will not be able to model nude effectively. The photographer shouldn't try to persuade her if she is shy or attaches some moral or social stigma to the project. Most likely, they will both regret the experience. Under no circumstances, should the model be tricked into a situation in which she will feel uncomfortable— although, even after she has agreed, it is frequently desirable to ease her into the full nude shot by beginning the shooting session with covering, progressing to seminude, and finally to the nude shots.

If the model is represented by an agency, it must be informed of the nature of the work prior to the model interview. Agencies know which girls are willing to do nude and seminude work and they also know that some models are insulted if

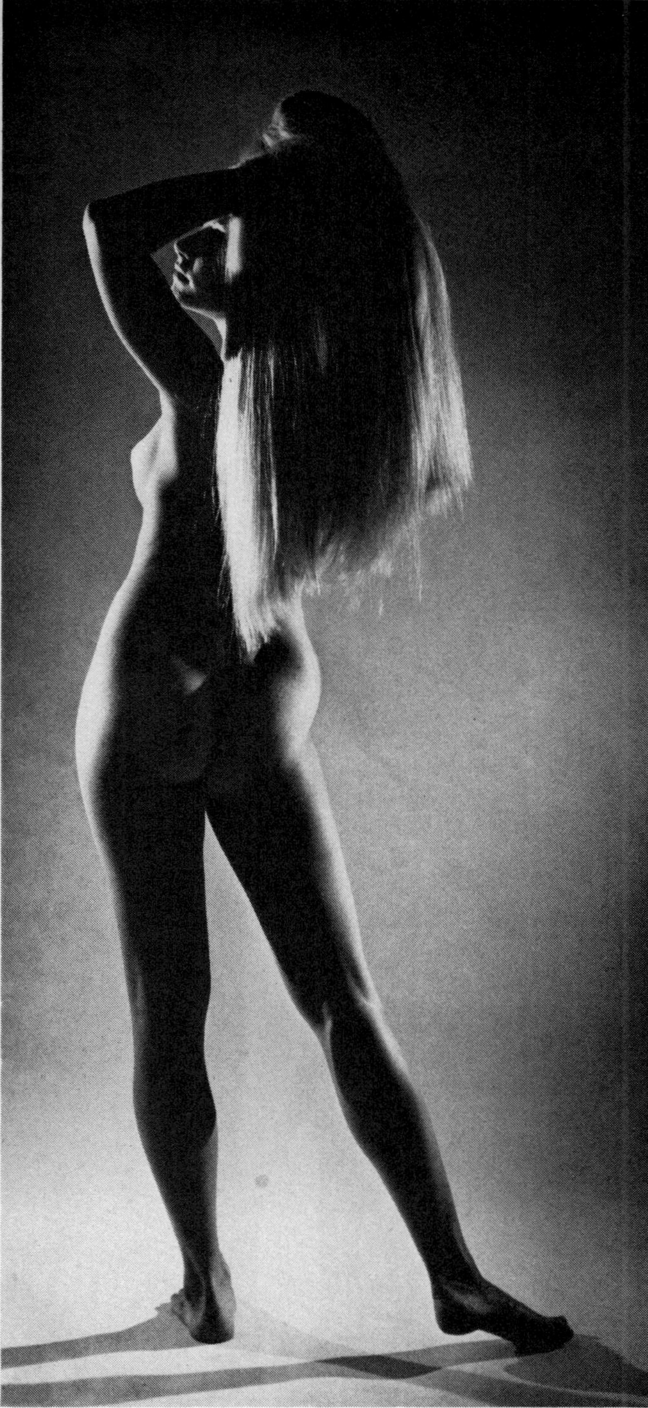

KAREN SNELL

The photographer should be careful to maintain the epitome of professional decorum while working with the nude model.

the photographer even broaches the subject.

Ideally, the photographer should avoid the subject totally with a model who is new to him unless, of course, she has been sent by the agency specifically to pose for a nude assignment. The professional nude model will have pictures to submit on the interview although final approval might involve her stripping to her underwear—and this part of the interview should be kept as brief and businesslike as possible.

If the model is required to undress for the interview, a dressing room and robe should be provided and the interview should involve only the photographer and possibly his client. Other persons in the studio should be warned to respect her privacy—even though a nude photograph of her will soon be published, she may not feel that in-person exposure is quite the same.

Once the model has been hired (and incidentally, that usually means double rates for professional models), careful arrangements should be made to make her as comfortable as possible. The dressing room of the professional should be equipped with body makeup, dressing robe and talc, as well as the usual makeup and hair supplies. Her privacy in the dressing room must be respected. The model should be cautioned to wear loose-fitting apparel to the assignment so valuable time isn't wasted waiting for her to lose flesh marks made by tight-fitting garments (and do be careful to have a nontextured, cushioned chair for her to sit on in the dressing room and in the studio—a cane-bottomed or rattan chair could be disastrous). Allow only qualified personnel to be present while shooting. People running in and out of the studio could quite justifiably annoy or embarrass her.

The photographer should be careful to maintain the epitome of professional decorum while working with her—ribald joking or an attitude that is too personal could backfire with a defensive model. □

what to look for

One of the most crucial decisions a photographer makes, in the type of photographic projects referred to in this book, is in the selection of the right model. It is a many-faceted decision—taking type, features, coloring, figure and personality into consideration. Perhaps the project determines the requirements of the model or, perhaps, the model inspires the project. Whichever the case, the end result must be harmonious and logical.

The physical appearance of the model, wardrobe, mood and position must combine artistically with the background, composition and lighting.

And, just as importantly, there must be a good communication and rapport between the photographer and his model. There is the right model for each situation; good casting is as important for a photographer as it is for a Broadway or motion picture producer.

The accompanying classification chart is offered as a general guide to types

of models and the way they are usually employed.

THE PHOTOGENIC GIRL

Frequently, a photographer deliberately chooses a subject who is a personality type that intrigues or amuses him or because of specific requirements of an assignment. These types can vary, of course, from child to grandparent, skinny to obese, tragic to comic.

More often; however, the delightful choice is that of an attractive, photogenic girl. Sadly, many photographers have learned that some girls who are very attractive in person don't seem as lovely when printed on a piece of paper—and occasionally, the reverse is true. A girl who might not be too impressive in person sometimes photographs surprisingly well.

It's a phenomenon that professional photographers are so aware of that they will rarely hire a model without seeing her portfolio. They well know the tricks the eyes can play. There are some fairly reliable standards, though. And, if a photographer is selecting a model without the aid of a professional model's portfolio, he can minimize his risks by judging certain features of his potential model.

Perhaps the most important facial feature is the nose. Small, narrow noses photograph the best. If a nose is somewhat wide and thick, it will be wider and thicker when flattened out on a piece of paper. A bump on the bridge of the nose can frequently catch a light and be magnified by the camera. Some improvement on imperfections can be achieved by special makeup techniques referred to in later chapters, but the degree of correction is limited.

If a model smiles, good teeth are a must. Many effective photos are made

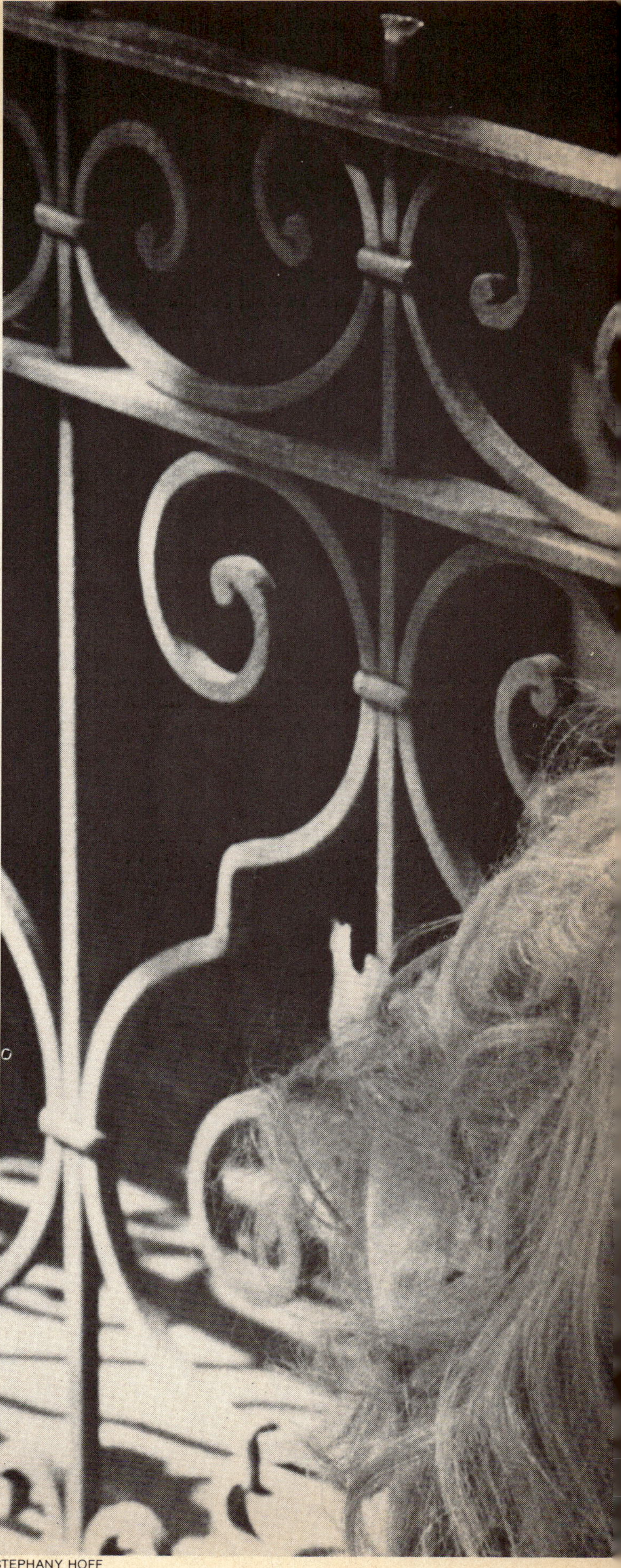

STEPHANY HOFF

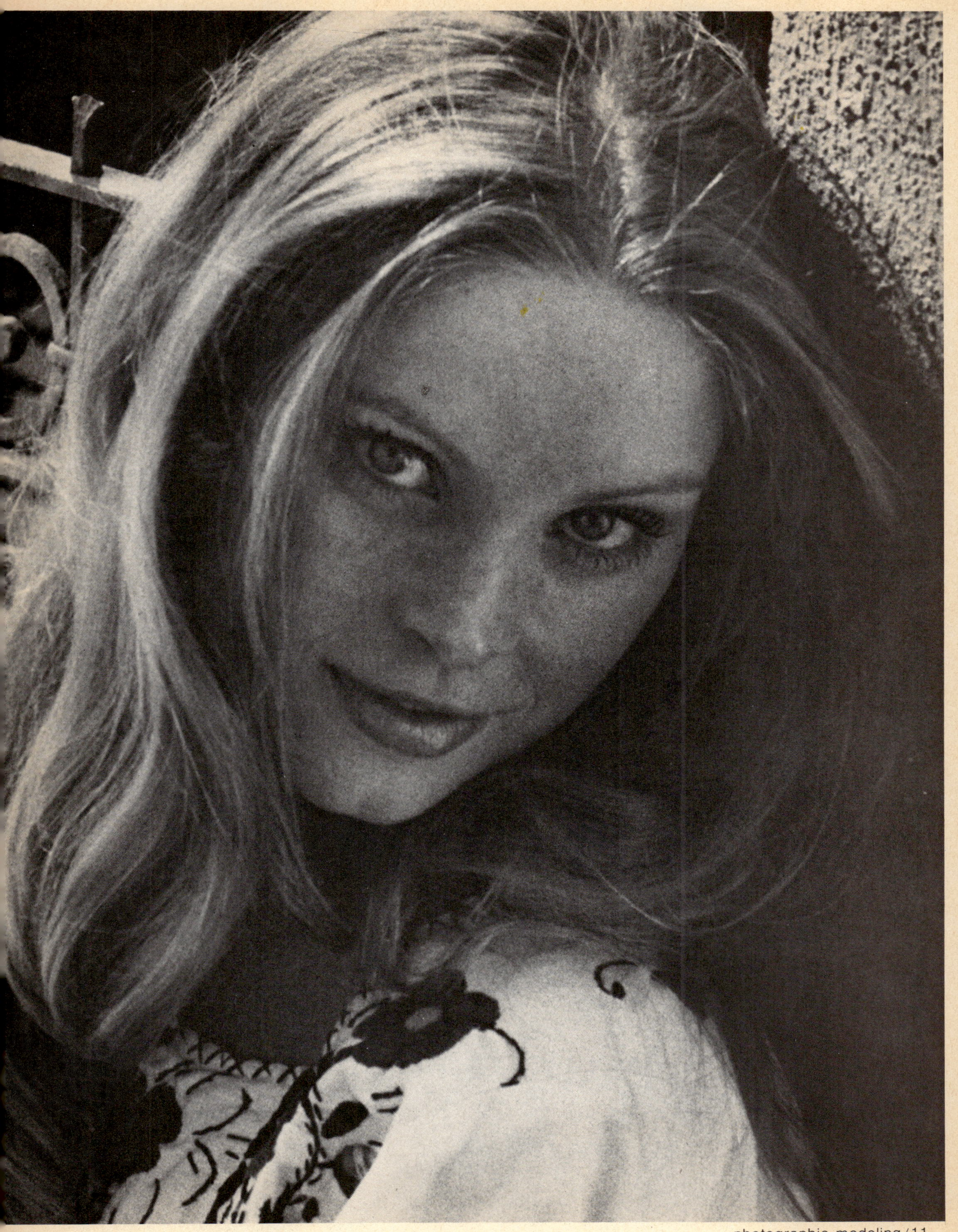

without full exposure of the teeth, but if a photographer chooses a model who has limitations in her expressions, he is deliberately crippling himself. Medium to large-size, straight teeth are best. Very small teeth or those that tend to tilt toward the inside of the mouth can be troublesome. Amazingly, some formations that are slightly bucktoothed can be quite photogenic—and many variations in formation might easily fall into the classification of individual beauty.

There is a trend away from *plastic prettiness* toward a more honest (and therefore broader) concept of beauty. It's a well-known fact that one of the most important models in the world has a sizable gap between her two front teeth. Unfortunately, this rather startling fact has encouraged a lot of girls with poor teeth to consider them unimportant and irrelevant to their photogenic potential. Actually, the particular model referred to usually covers the gap with a slip-on insert between the two front teeth. It was only after she had attained considerable fame that her dental secret was exposed and, in addition, this inspiring model is utterly beautiful and superbly talented in front of the camera.

Photographers should be cautious also of overly thick or thin lips—and do observe your model on your initial interview and watch to see if she smiles easily and freely or if she has a tendency to fight her smile and pull the muscles down at the corners of her mouth.

Eyes are the easiest of all to enhance with makeup but they are also an extremely important feature. Large, well-spaced eyes are the most photogenic. The model's eyebrows shouldn't dominate her face. They should be well shaped and soft in effect. The wrong makeup techniques here can ruin your photos faster than any other cosmetic area, so do counsel your model in what you require of her and have her study the makeup techniques in this book.

Complicated filters, lighting and makeup cannot completely disguise a poor complexion. It's an important factor to consider. Professional models are usually careful about too much sun exposure. Sunburns and tans can photograph blotchy, dry and tend to accentuate lines.

Traditionally, the oval face has been considered the perfect shape. There have been, however, terrifically successful models with heart-shaped, round or square faces. And hair styles can often soften extremes in these facial shapes. The structure that has planes and shadows created by strong cheek bones and hollows in the cheeks is certainly much more exciting to photograph than a fleshy face that tends to catch light uniformly and results in a flat effect, rather than an illusion of depth.

The photogenic girl also has a flattering hair style (or, hopefully, styles). Every great model is an artist with her own hair. Dyed black hair or over-bleached blondes can create super lighting problems and hard effects. And dark roots on girls who should pay a visit to the hair colorist will definitely show up in your camera, so don't bother to waste your film.

Cameras tend to shorten and widen the body so slim, tall girls grace most model agencies. Whatever her height, it's vital that the model is trim, firm and well proportioned. Flat tummies and firm thighs are super important. The clever model can minimize and maximize the rest of herself with amazing results.

Perhaps even more important than facial or bodily structure, there is a kind of inner magic the truly photogenic model possesses. There is an indefinable aura of confidence, beauty of spirit, enthusiasm and warmth. Call it charisma, if you will, or personal magnetism; the good model always projects a very special quality that sets her apart from the ordinary girl.

CREATING THE MODEL LOOK

The natural or born model usually has a certain amount of good instinct about the way she should look. But, for a truly professional effect, those instincts usually need to be developed and guided toward creating the perfect, special, unique look or image of the individual model. Ideally, she should never try to create a poor carbon copy of some other, perhaps already established, model. It's important to respect the extraordinary individuality of each model. Then, determine the hairstyle, makeup and general effect that enhances her and creates a positive identity within the current fashion framework.

In order to be effective in guiding your model toward her own ideal look, it's a good idea for both the photographer and the model to thoroughly acquaint themselves with current trends in fashion, makeup and hairstyling. Existing trends in the latest magazines should be studied—with the understanding that fashions are an expression of the times—economically, socially and even politically. The effect will not be acceptable unless it is synchronized to the times and there is always a look, within this framework, that can be developed to flatter and enhance the model without sacrificing her individuality.

Of course, a model must feel comfortable with the look that is decided upon. If she feels it conflicts in any way with her own personality or concept of herself, the result will be synthetic and unconvincing.

This particular phase of a model's development requires a great deal of understanding from the consulting photographer and an even greater understanding of the model herself to the point where she can release old concepts of herself that might delay her from fully blossoming into her own special kind of beauty.

All agencies, stylists and photographers have been annoyed and frustrated by misguided creatures who have ruined themselves with a cheap, too-theatrical effect, or a look that is not related to their own age group. These people are particularly difficult to advise or direct.

It's a real delight to view a model who knows herself and seems to like what she knows and has developed expertise and originality in her presentation of herself. □

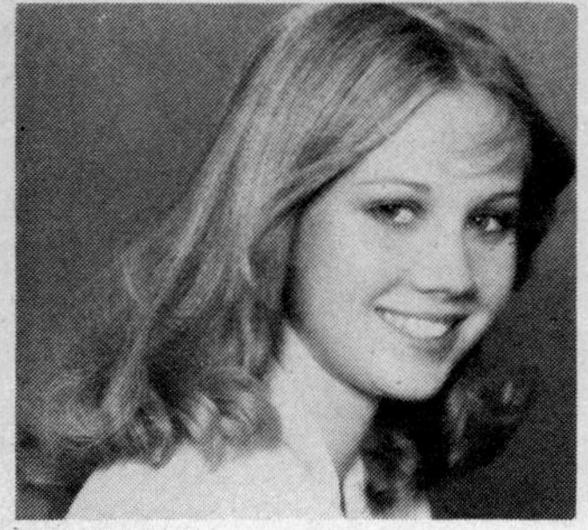

CARINA HAILEY

'TEEN MODEL

Age Range—13 to 19.

Height—5' to 5'10".

Size—All junior sizes.

Personality—Cute, fresh, happy, vivacious, innocent.

Identified With—*'Teen Magazine* covers.

Special Features and Notes—Not necessarily used in fashion work—she's fresher and less stylized and sophisticated than the Junior fashion model. Does magazine covers, *'Teen Magazine* editorial sections, product shots.

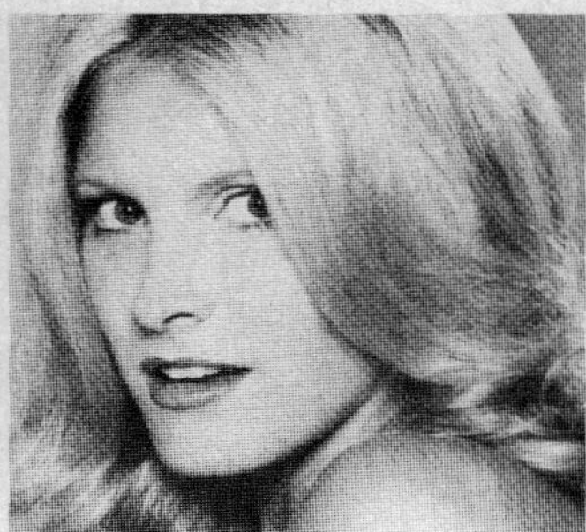

GAIL HEWITT

JUNIOR/YOUNG FASHION MODEL

Age Range—14 to 22/17 to 25 or older, perhaps.

Height—5'5" to 5'10".

Size—5, 6, 7, 8, 9, 10.

Personality—Has a young *in* expression, moderately sophisticated, confident, can be serious or vivacious, rather friendly and pleasant.

Identified With—*Seventeen, McCalls* fashions, *Ladies Home Journal, Glamour, Charm,* some TV.

Special Features and Notes—This is a very positive *look,* somewhat sophisticated but only in the sense that is totally acceptable in the 'teen world.

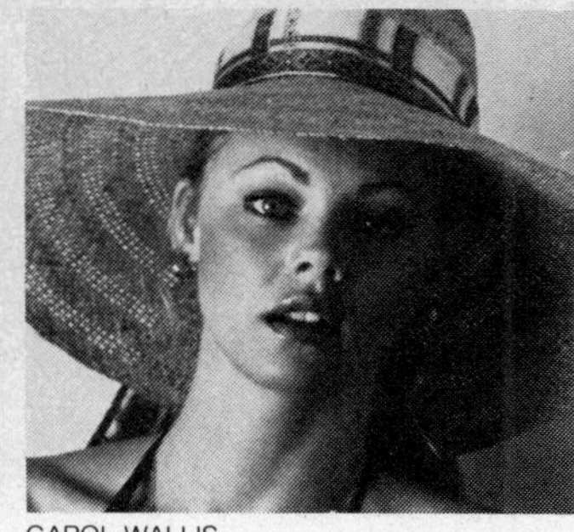

CAROL WALLIS

HIGH FASHION

Age Range—18 to 28 or older, perhaps.

Height—5'7" to 6'.

Size—6, 8, 10.

Personality—Haughty, highly sophisticated, utterly confident.

Identified With—*Harper's Bazaar, Vogue.*

Special Features and Notes—An absolutely *positive* look, extreme makeup and hairstyling, highly stylized poses, more popular in New York market than in other modeling areas.

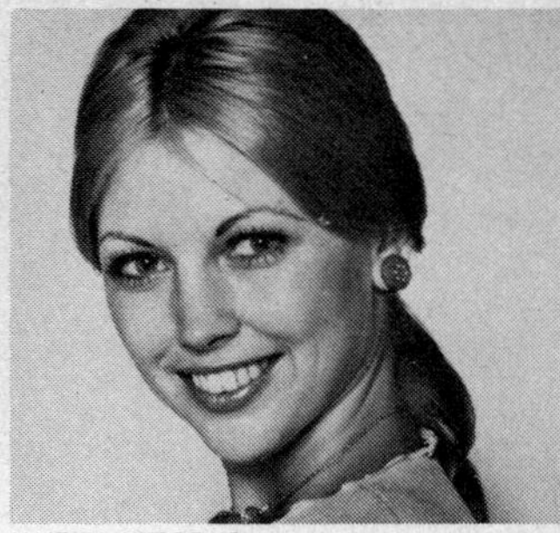

JANEEN ANDERSON

YOUNG HOUSEWIFE

Age Range—19 to 28.

Height—5'4" to 5'8" or 5'9".

Size—6, 7, 8, 9, 10.

Personality—Friendly, wholesome, pleasant, happy.

Identified With—Product and advertising shots.

Special Features and Notes—Moderate makeup and hairstyling—doesn't seem to pose at all. Pretty but not highly stylized—could be a young fashion model toned down.

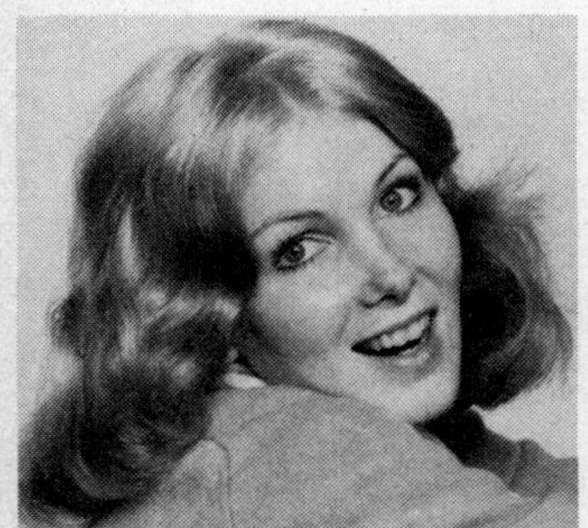

NANCI ROBERTS COWSILL

PRETTY COVER GIRL

Age Range—14 to 22.

Height—Not a factor.

Size—Figure sometimes not a factor.

Personality—Outdoor girl, pretty, wholesome, happy.

Identified With—Magazine covers, billboards, product advertising.

Special Features and Notes—Beautiful face, perfect complexion, engaging smile, pretty hair—usually longish.

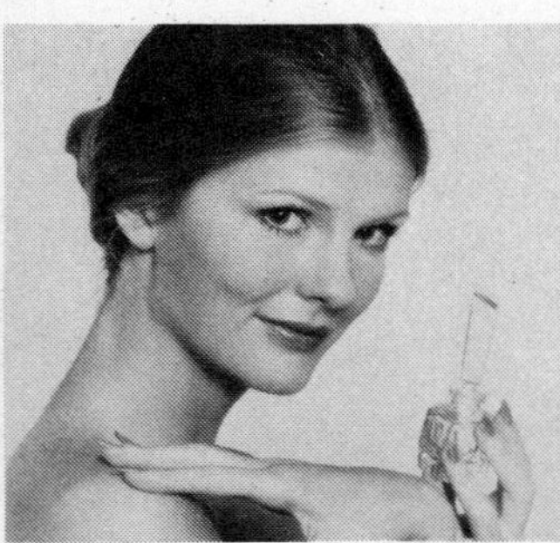

TAMARA BOWES

HOUSEWIFE OR YOUNG MATRON

Age Range—26 to 40.

Height—5'4" to 5'7".

Size—6, 8, 10, 12, 14

Personality—Wholesome, mature, competent, pleasant, happy.

Identified With—Product advertising shots, some fashion in women's home magazines.

Special Features and Notes—Slice-of-life types. Must not look like a model, a real-life lady next door.

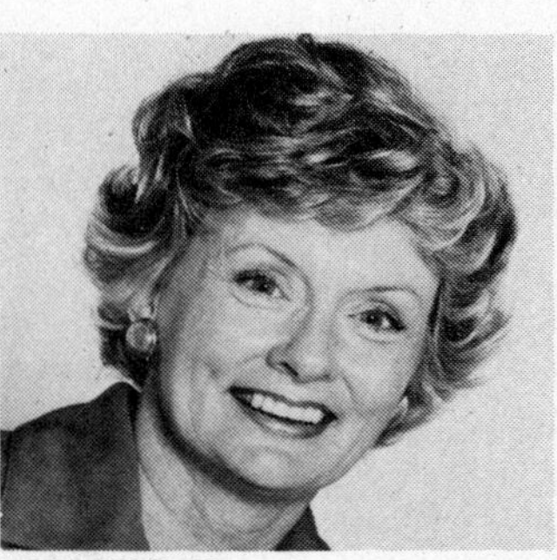

RHODA DESOMER

MATRONS/GRANDMOTHERS

Age Range—Mature, 40 and over.

Height—5'4" to 5'7"—rarely over unless grande dame or dowager type.

Size—Any reasonable proportions.

Personality—Motherly, pleasant, happy. Comes in all lovable types—wizened and fragile, plump and jolly.

Identified With—Product advertising.

Special Features and Notes—Same as for Young Housewife/Matron, or she might be a *grand lady* type, must be lovable.

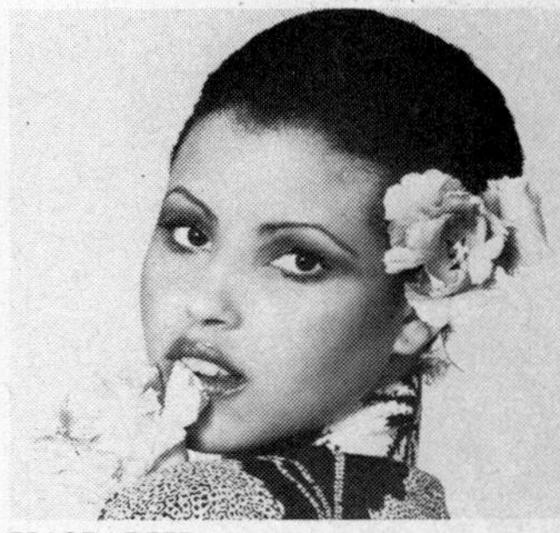

TRACEY FIFER

ETHNIC

Age Range—All ages.

Height—Depends on the assignment.

Size—Depends on the assignment.

Personality—Can be serious or vivacious depending on age and type.

Identified With—Product advertising, fashion and covers.

Special Features and Notes—There are more opportunities than ever in this field though professional preparation is necessary as with other types.

how
to
pose

Experienced photographers and models alike generally agree that great models have an innate instinct about what to do in front of the camera.

The born model instinctively moves with grace and a natural awareness of how she looks in the camera lens. She also has natural acting ability and the ability to express a great variety of moods.

But even natural born models need a basic framework of fundamental techniques and, once a photographer discovers such a girl, it is well worth the time and effort it takes to help her whenever possible to learn these fundamentals so she can express herself freely in front of the camera with sure, professional results.

There is much ground to cover before the model actually gets in front of a camera. The photographer and model alike can learn a great deal about body movements, interpretation of fashion, facial expressions, lines and angles and much, much more by the introduction of two major study techniques.

First of all, you need to become acquainted with the current trends in photographic modeling techniques. Along with fashion (partly because of varying fashion needs), posing techniques vary from one fashion era to the next.

If one were to study old fashion magazines it would be easy to recognize marked differences in body movements, leg positions,

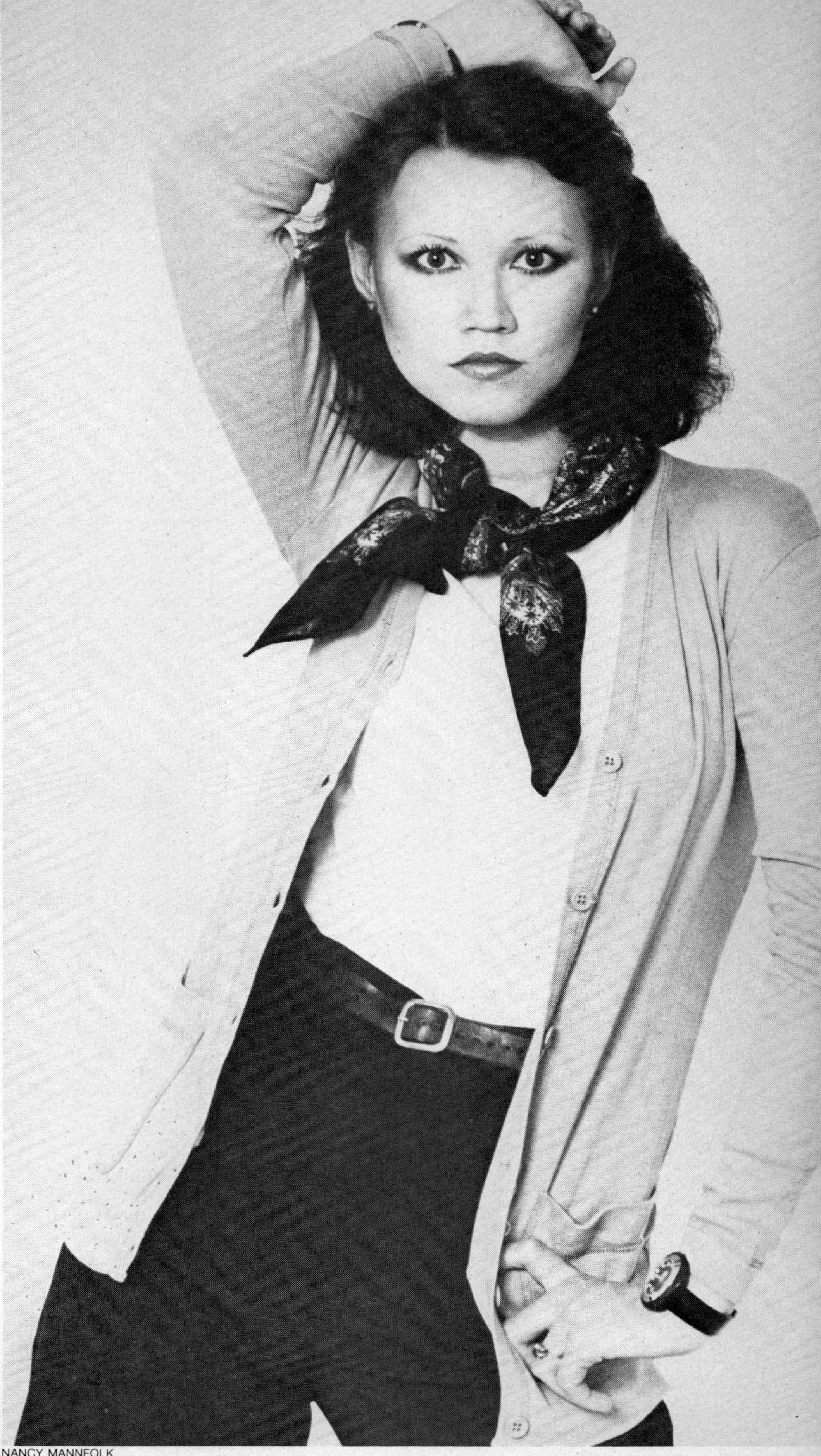

NANCY MANNFOLK

even facial expressions between today's techniques and those of three, five or 10 years ago. So, first, the model should get a feeling for the current looks and techniques.

Generally, a woman flips through a fashion magazine in a rather casual manner, pausing occasionally to enjoy a particular picture or take note of an attractive design. But she rarely stops to analyze all that went into creating each picture.

The novice model and photographer should approach a fashion magazine as a textbook with each page a challenge to be analyzed and used as a step in learning.

Go through good fashion magazines with your protégée model and point out different leg positions, different gestures, facial expressions and body angles. Look for standing, sitting, and reclining positions and point out how the model relates to the clothes she is wearing and the background she is posing against. Note how props are held and how multi-model poses are arranged. Show her how to determine major light sources and how the model uses these to her advantage.

After the model has studied the magazines and the following chapters, she is ready to attempt the second phase of her study program in front of a full-length mirror. Encourage her to practice at home alone in front of the mirror—first emulating poses she likes to relate to in the fashion

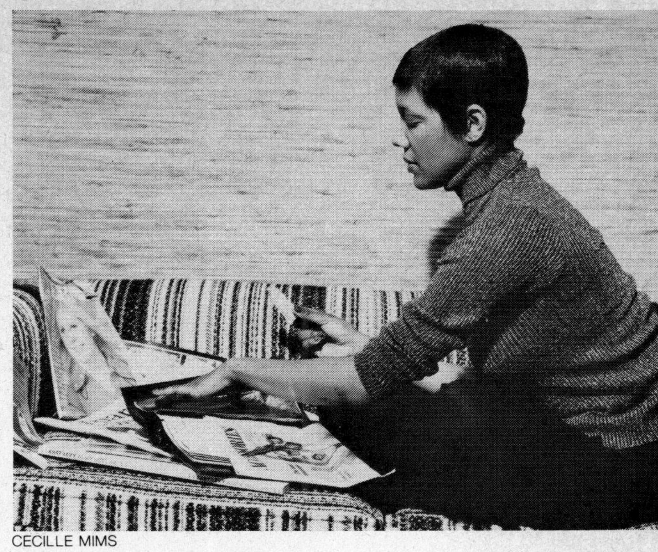

CECILLE MIMS

Would-be model should keep a scrapbook of magazine pictures she likes, go over the pictures with her photographer, and keep notes on their observations.

magazine and then creating her own poses. Then, have her work in front of the mirror while you watch so she will become accustomed to being free and expressive with an audience, and learn to take directions as you help her to perfect and refine her poses.

These learning steps can be effectively augmented by encouraging the model to create a scrapbook of pictures she likes. She can look at pictures for hours, but those shots will belong to the model and photographer who shot them until she makes a tangible effort to bring them into the scope of her own experience by cutting out the picture and making notes that include your and her observations regarding the shots. The following pages will serve as a guideline to your model's learning experience.

FACIAL EXPRESSIONS

Turning on an expression is not quite as easy as switching on an electric light bulb. An emotional preparation must be made. The expression is a result of a feeling—teach your model that her expression is the

effect, not the cause, and the cause (feeling) must come first. She should learn to mentally isolate herself into a private little "thought-area" island.

Experiment with the novice model—have her lower her head and *think* the feeling very hard until she experiences the feeling so thoroughly that she can't hold it back any longer. Then, have her lift her head and let it all come out at once. At first, the change from mood to mood may take a few minutes; later, she'll be able to make mood changes in a matter of seconds.

It's important that you express approval during her first experiments with mood changes—she's exposing emotions which the world has taught her to hide and she'll need to gain confidence in herself and in you.

One of the primary means we have of conveying a variety of emotions and reactions is our facial expressions. Even with the aid of verbal communication, we still depend upon facial expression to witness for words being used. In still photography, the model is deprived of the aid of verbal communication. She must tell her story with her face. And, at the same time, must appeal as a uniquely beautiful personality.

Most of us have had the unpleasant experience, at one time or another, of having our facial expression misinterpreted by another (one is being thoughtful and accused of being unhappy). It is now of special importance that the model learns to communicate an accurate message through her facial expressions. The model must learn that a photographer's camera is an incredibly perceptive device, and is very quick to record an insincere expression. *The expression must always be backed up by an emotion* no matter how fleeting the moment may be—during the precise split second when the exposure is made, the model must be actually feeling what her face is trying to say.

Sincerity, unfortunately, is not always enough. Besides feeling an emotion and effectively showing the same facially, the model is required to do this as attractively as possible, avoiding any facial distortions and, at the same time, concealing imperfections. For instance, a strong laugh must not reveal the gums above the teeth, or the eyes must not be crinkled into a slit. The expression must, of course, be convincing but it should also have a special personality of its own—it should be provocative, enchanting, enigmatic, sensitive, exciting, interesting, mischievous, sexy—it must have a quality which evokes a definite response in the viewer.

SMILING—One of the most important expressions is the smile. (Encourage your model to use it often in front of and away from the camera.) A model's smile, whether it is a very slight smile, a grin or a full smile, must be perfected to the greatest degree possible. The smile, more than any other expression, must be spontaneous. Because of the disarming nature of the expression, an insincere smile seems to be regarded as an ultimate in deceit and people are inclined to react very strongly against it.

A photographer's model has to know how to express a genuine smile at any given moment—and that can be very difficult. Try it yourself, right now—not easy, is it? Even experienced models might find it a challenge while freezing on a location beach shot at dawn or sweltering under hot lights in furs at the end of a day when the photographer and his crew begin to become tense and difficult.

And beyond the concerns of being spontaneous and real, the model has to determine what degree of smile is appropriate. Obviously, a full smile might not be appropriate in a tender shot of a mother holding a baby to her breast and, conversely, the Madonna-like smile won't do on a roller coaster.

The model must also concern herself with keeping her face pretty. Some girls find that a very full smile results in a puffiness under the eyes, or too many crinkles in the corners at the temples. Sometimes the gums above the teeth are unattractively exposed. Many models have to correct a tendency to smile crookedly and learn not to pull down at the corners of the mouth. There are some mouths that become too strained in the upper lip in a full smile and a pulled crescent wrinkle forms above the upper lip. A smile that tends to be so tight that the lips seem to

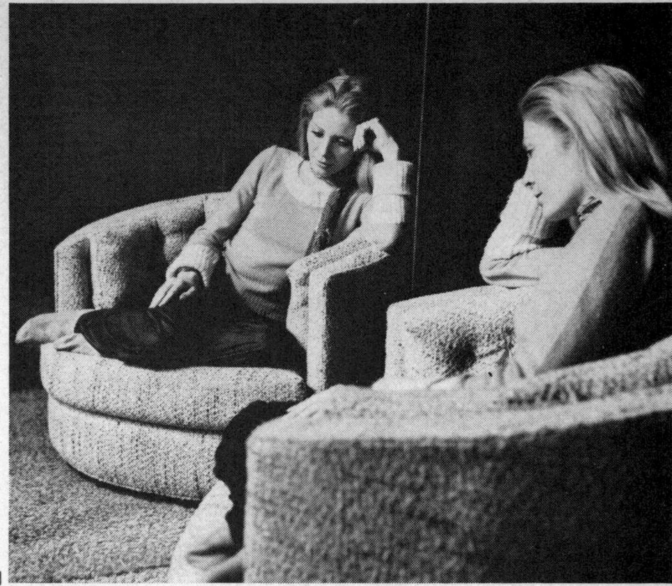

JON MARLOW

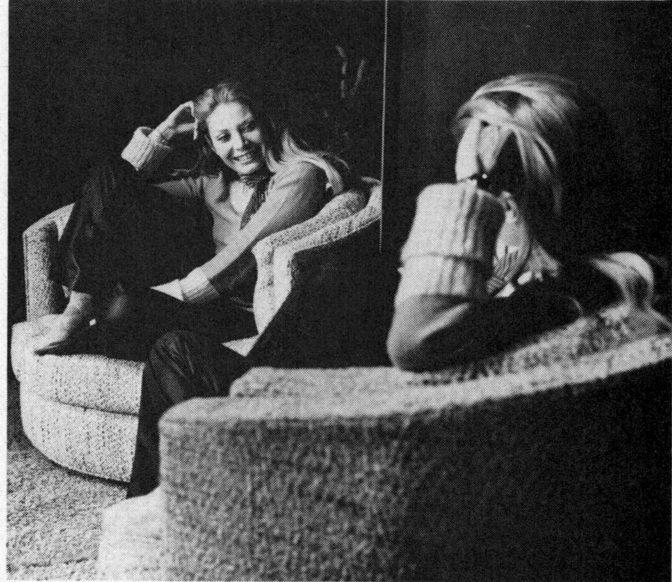

disappear can be a real problem. Hopefully, all a photographer will need to do is to compliment and praise his model's smile—call her "happy face" or something similar—or use some other method to let the model know that her smile is exceptionally appealing.

If the novice model is really having a difficult time, it might help to sit down with her in front of the mirror and help her practice perfecting her smile. He can show her which smiles he considers the prettiest and tactfully suggest habits she should avoid.

Harsh criticism in this area could permanently cripple the model—at least in working with the photographer who has embarrassed her—so take it easy, both in the practice sessions and especially behind the camera.

Encourage your model to relax her lips as much as possible in her smile. Unless the model is deliberately striving for an impish, mischievous effect in which the lips might become more tensed, the lips should be kept loose with the cheeks doing most of the work.

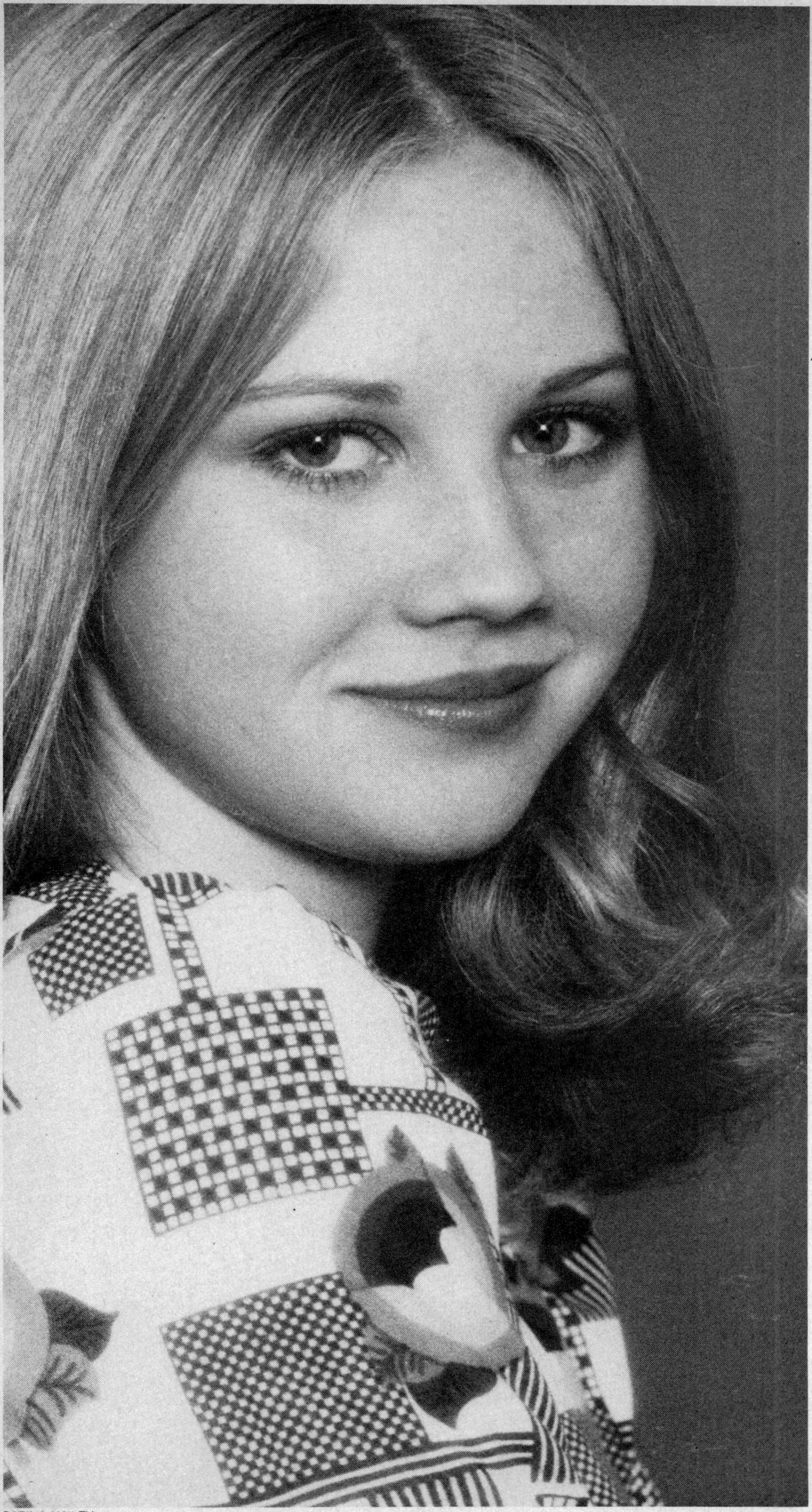

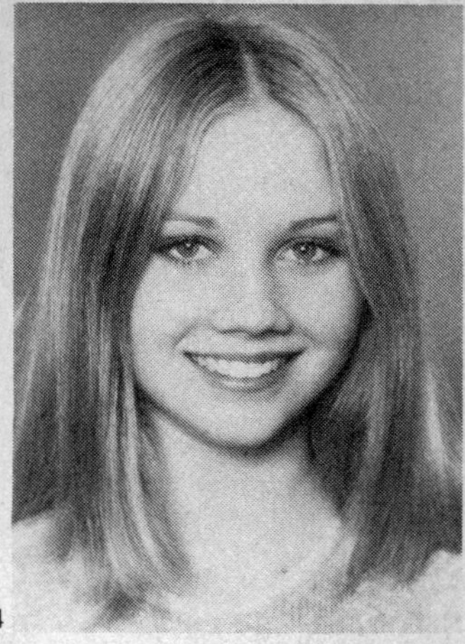

4

1, 2. Model's expression must be preceded by a feeling. Have model lower her head and think the feeling very hard, then lift her head and let it all come out. Mirror lets her see how successful her expression is.
3. Closed-mouth smile can convey moods from impishness to sweetness to sexiness.
4. One of the most important expressions is the smile, and it must be perfected to the greatest degree possible.

Get her to try every degree of smile possible, starting out with just a pleasant, closed mouth tiny suggestion of a smile, gradually increasing to a big smile that fully exposes all of the front upper teeth. (Very few girls look well showing the lower teeth in a smile—an out-and-out laugh, sometimes, but not always, might show both the upper and lower teeth.)

The novice model should try these smiles many times in mirror practice. One little experiment will not be enough. After both of you are satisfied with every degree of smile, she should then combine her efforts with eye expression.

The eyes should be kept wide open and sparkling with expression in smiling

CARINA HAILEY

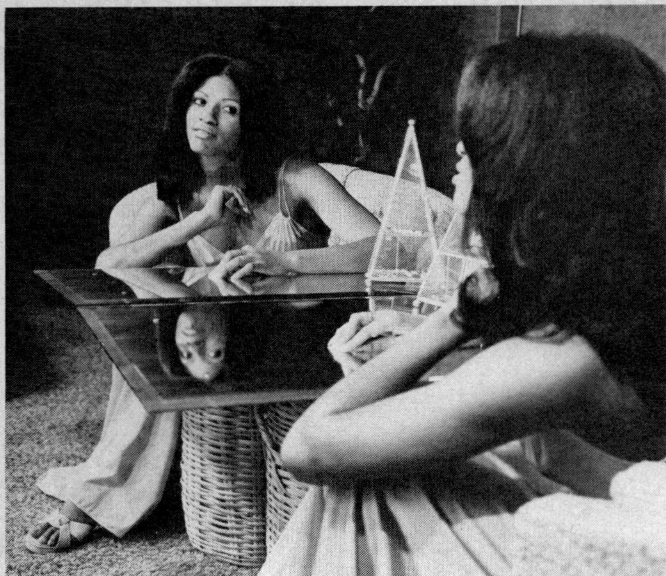

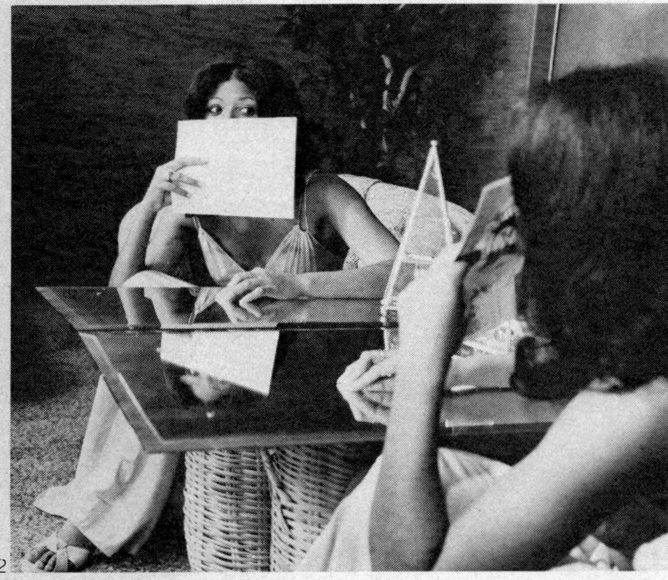

1. 2. The eyes can tell the story. To learn how to "talk with her eyes," model should practice in front of mirror, thinking of a word or phrase, then expressing thought with eyes. Covering lower portion of face during this excercise can help.
3. Model has to become totally unaware of camera or anyone around her to reflect subtle pensive mood.

The moods of a closed mouth smile can vary from impish to sweetness to sexiness. Search through some magazines with the novice model so she can understand the range of moods possible.

MOUTH SLIGHTLY OPEN—When people are totally unself-conscious and truly concentrating upon someone or something, they often leave their mouths slightly open. The special charm of this expression is the effect that the model is totally unaware of herself—completely absorbed in a mood or thought. A variety of results might be achieved—a high fashion model might assume a very haughty effect, a glamour type might look sexy and the junior model might present an extremely vulnerable, little girl effect.

LAUGHING—Some of the best moments in life are those that provoke unrestrained laughter, and some of the best pictures are the result. It takes practice to learn to be so uninhibited at a moment's notice but it is an emotional high that a good model should be able to reach easily.

If your model is restrained, encourage her to actually break out into real vocal laughter. Laugh along with her if necessary. Even a silent laugh has to be accompanied by natural diaphragm involvement. It must happen to seem real. Also note how short bursts of air are released from the mouth, even in a silent laugh. If the model doesn't master this, you're more likely to get a picture that looks like she's yawning.

Your model should be encouraged to practice various degrees of laughter from the pretty laugh with enough restraint to avoid crinkly eyes and distorted features to the laugh where everything is let go, like you might catch when a cold ocean wave breaks over her. Many photographers try to instill a candid effect in their work so it appears the model has been caught off guard in

practice sessions. Note: A truly beautiful smile requires nice teeth—a slightly chipped tooth may need to be filed to a smooth edge or a slip-on cap fitted by her dentist might disguise an unfortunate separation.

CLOSED SMILES—Not all smiles look like toothpaste advertisements. Some of the nicest smiles are completely unadorned by the teeth. Many models find the closed mouth smile rather difficult to master. Pleasant thoughts, lively eyes and lots of mirror practice should do the trick.

the middle of a living situation. This slice-of-life effect is much easier for a viewer to relate to and it brings action and believability to the shot.

It would be boring, indeed, to flip through every magazine and find all the models smiling or laughing at you. People just don't do that all the time. But there is one thing most photographers will tell you that many younger girls do a lot, and that is, talk. Many effective pictures are shot with the model looking as though she were actually saying something at the moment the camera shutter fired.

Some models prefer actual vocalization of a word though most can achieve a believable effect by whispering the word. Using a word helps the model's face come alive. No expression is a matter of lip formation alone; it must have meaning behind it.

PENSIVE MOODS— Expressions involving lots of animation can sometimes be easier to get from a model than the quieter, more subtle expressions which reflect a contemplative, pensive, more private mood. In these instances, the model has to become totally unaware of the camera or anyone around her. She seems to be lost in thought. There is a fine line of difference between a pensive and a sullen expression. The photographer must encourage the model to retain sweetness in her expression.

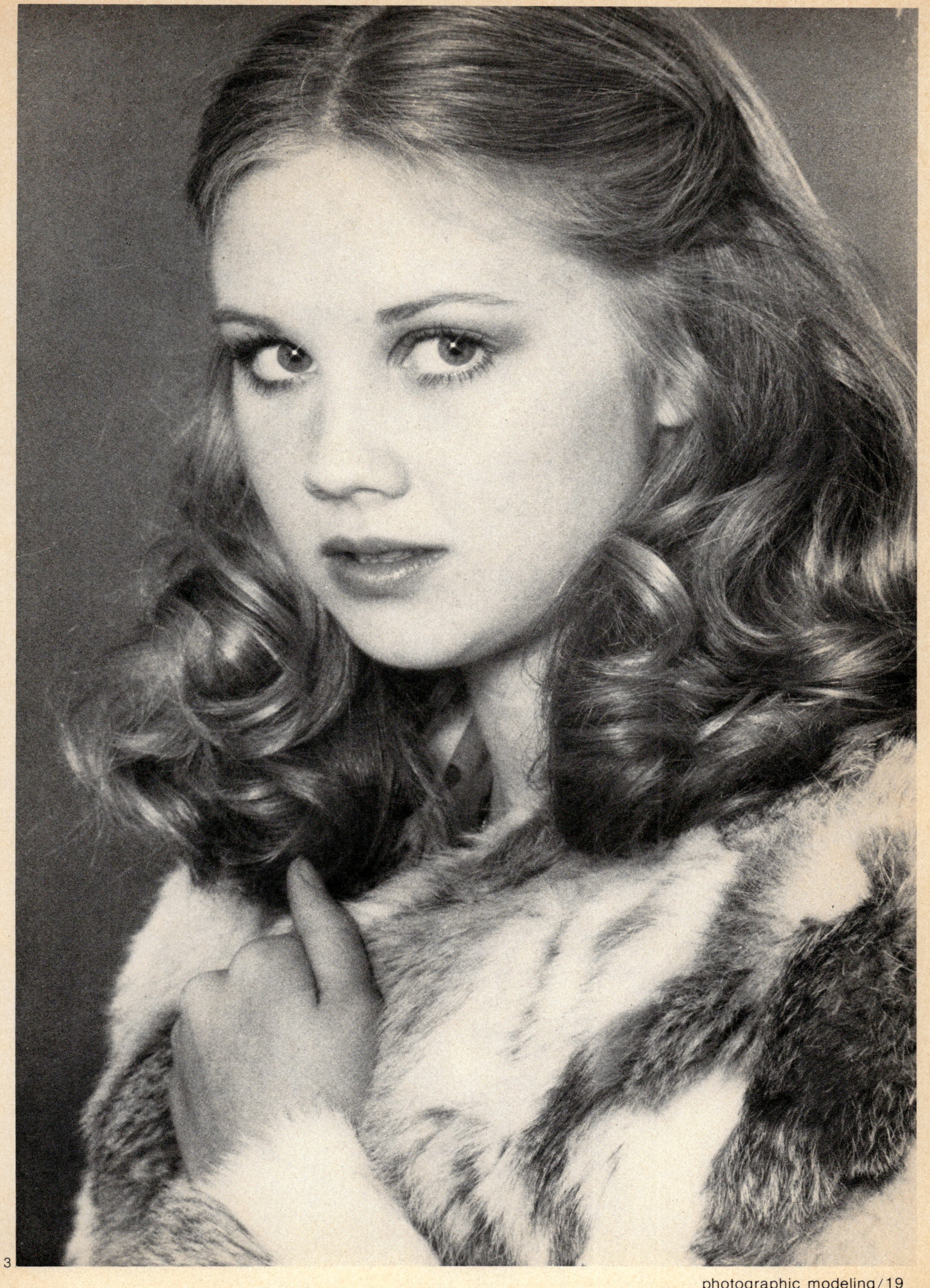

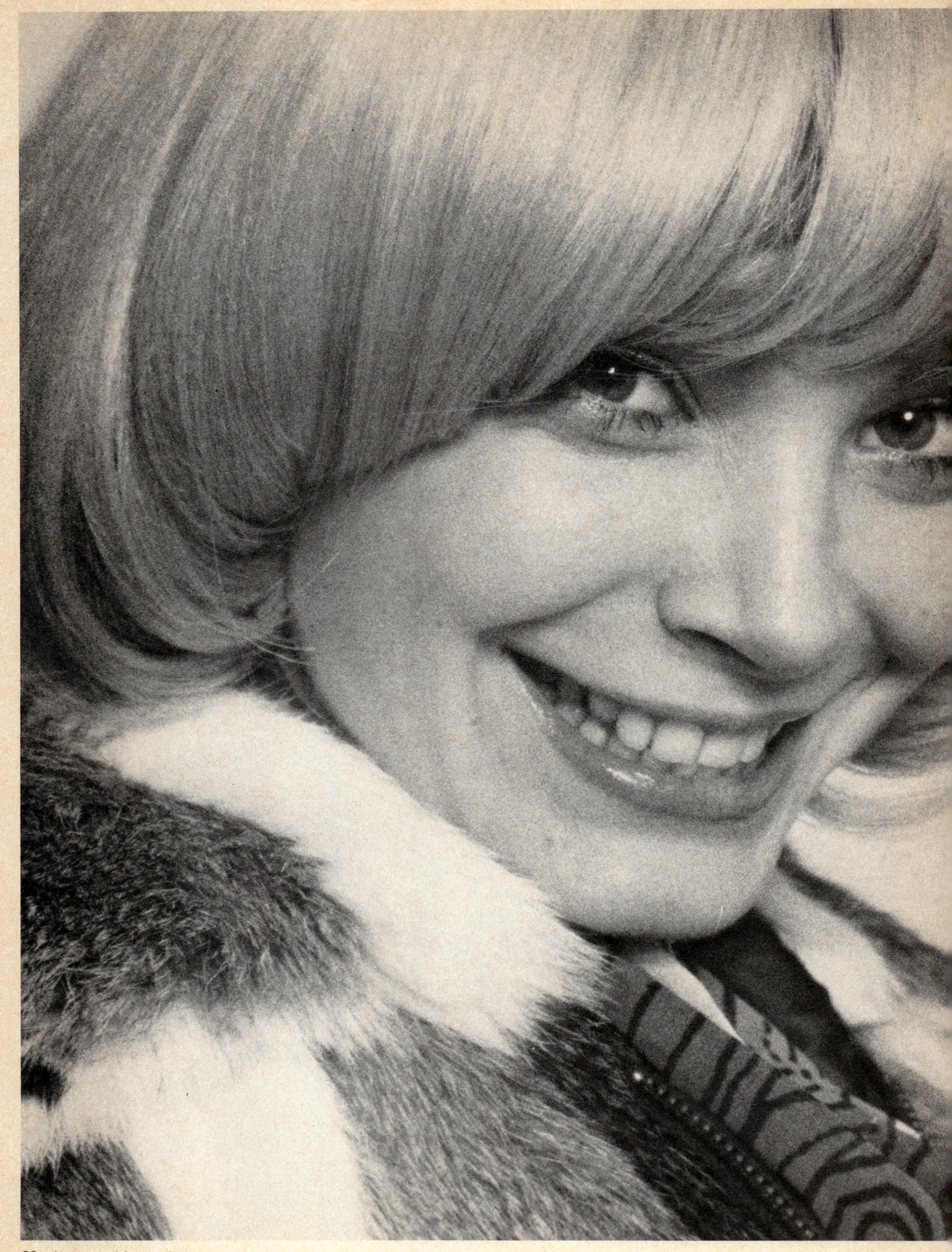

EYE EXPRESSIONS—It's very easy (and often disastrous) for a novice model to just stare with her eyes—no life, no sparkle, no meaning. Expressive eyes are a vital ingredient in an exciting picture, and the model must learn, along with the photographer, to time the peak of her eye expression to the release of the shutter.

It's nearly impossible to sustain real live expression in the eyes for a matter of minutes. It takes a great deal of practice and concentration to sustain eye expression even for three seconds. Most models lower their eyes a bit to rest them (especially helpful in bright sunlight or under incandescent lighting) right before the shot and then look up with the desired, spontaneous expression.

The photographer should watch for the moment when her eye focuses—and yet, try to catch it before the expression begins to fade. If a photographer finds his novice model unable to effectively master the art of eye expression, he can help her by sitting in front of a mirror with her and teaching her how to "talk with her eyes." She should lower her head, think a phrase or a word, then express the thought with her eyes without saying a word. If her eyes are still dead, have her cover the lower portion of her face and practice until the eyes tell the whole story.

Additionally, the photographer should watch her carefully in order to anticipate the peak of the expression he is looking for. There is nothing as frustrating to novice or pro model alike than to work up to the desired feeling and expression only to find the photographer asleep at the

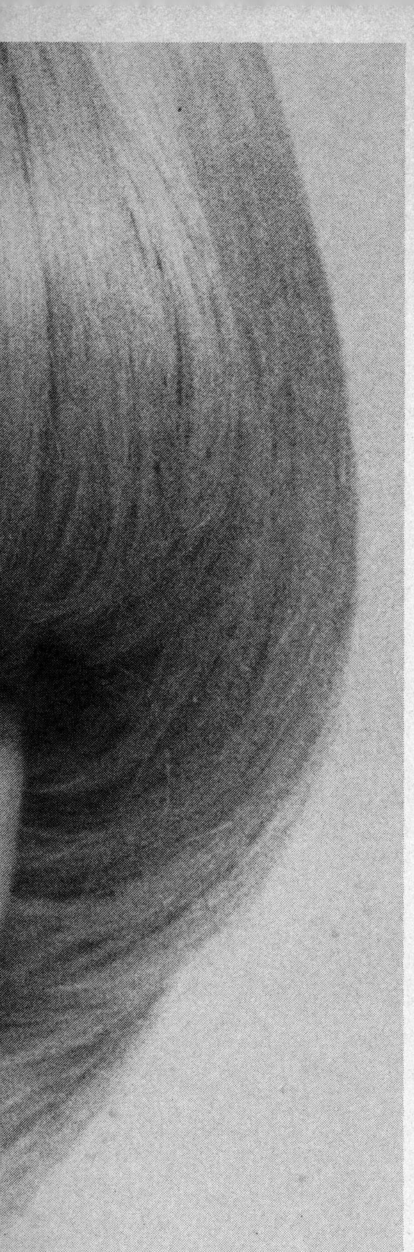

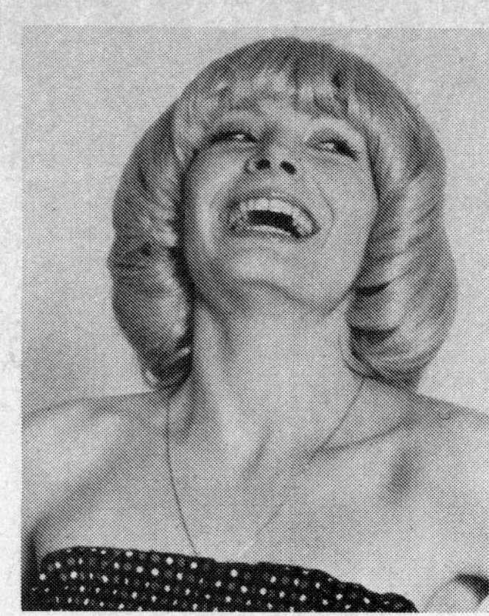

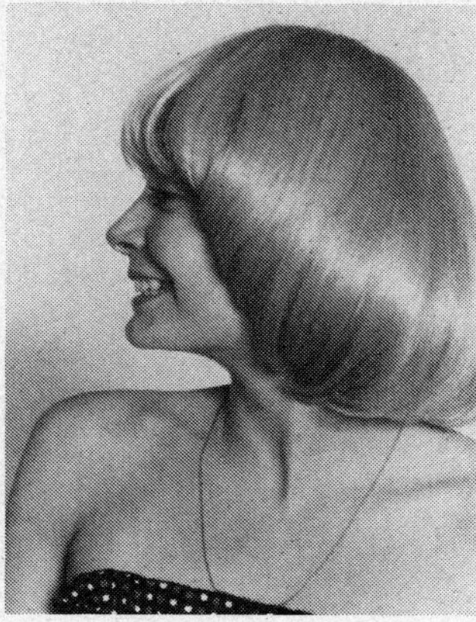

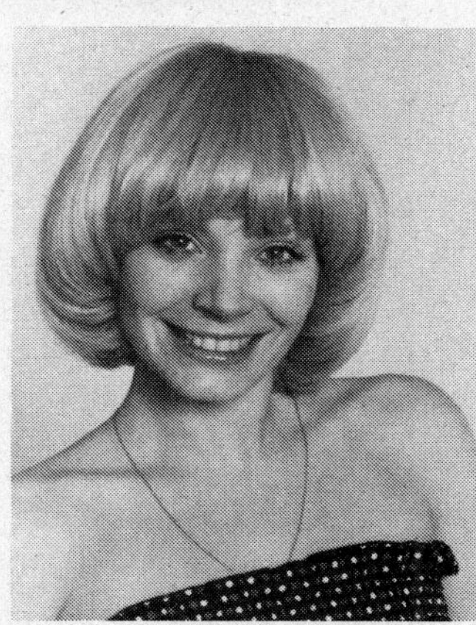

It is not always necessary to look full face at camera. Model should become aware of freedom of facial angles as well as eye direction available to her.

trigger and miss the shot because he wasn't quick enough to catch it.

EYE FOCUS—Even if a model believes her expression, the effect can still look much like a stare if she has failed to focus her eyes properly. The pupils change visibly when a person is looking out way beyond the horizon and then looks at a close object.

Experiment with eye focus by trying to look through and beyond the furthest wall in the room—now look at the wall (preferably a picture on the wall), then look at something halfway across the room; then at a very close object at the same eye level. Do you feel how your eyes adjust?

Try this experiment with your model—she will soon learn that she can ruin a photo by not focusing her eyes properly just as quickly as you can if you don't focus your camera.

This eye adjustment is visible to the camera—and the photographer should encourage the model to imagine that she is looking at, smiling at or talking to someone or something right off camera. On the other hand, she might very well be looking at a broad expanse of scenery that would involve a different horizon-viewed eye focus.

The application of these techniques soon becomes quite automatic to a model but, at first, it is important that she understand that unfocused eyes will not generally create a totally believable effect.

The model should understand that it is not always necessary to look full face at the camera. Show her examples of ¾ angles, profiles, chin tilted up or down, head tilted to one side or the other so that she can become aware of the freedom of facial angles as well as eye direction available to her.

JON MARLOW

The model can look up, down or sideways—generally, if she is looking up, above lens level, she should be looking at something specific, usually established in the photo. Otherwise, your model might look like she's praying, or worse, rolling her eyes. Even with an established justification for looking upward, some models don't look very good looking up under the eyebrows with a lot of white showing beneath the pupils. Looking away from the camera at an extreme angle can also be a problem, especially if the whites of the eyes are all that is visible to the camera and the model looks as though she has no pupils at all.

Nevertheless, the model should be encouraged to direct her attention away from the camera as well as toward it for variations in mood and effect. □

THE STANCE

When a novice model starts to pose for her first full-length pictures, her initial concern is invariably what she should do with her feet. ''How should I stand?'' she will usually lament. A basic knowlege of fundamental stances will help her build confidence. Soon, she learns that there are actually a limitless number of leg and feet positions. But, at first, it won't help to tell her to stand any way she wants—she will feel more secure with a basic stance or one of it's variations.

THE BASIC STANCE—Instruct the model to stand facing the camera. Draw an imaginary line for her from the model to the camera. The model should then stand on one foot (either left or right) with the toe pointing on a line of about 45 degrees from the camera to body line. This foot can be identified as the basic foot. The other foot (which should be identified as the free foot) should be placed with the heel about two inches in front of the instep of the basic foot with the toe pointing straight to the camera.

The position of the feet is not the entire story. The whole body should become involved. Shoulders should be in a line which is more or less square (perpendicular) to the camera-body line, and the hips should be twisted away from the camera with the back hip and basic foot corresponding.

The body's weight will be placed on the basic (or back) foot and hip. Thus an optical illusion is created in which the model's shoulders look broad, waist looks tiny, and the hips are diminished in size.

VARIATIONS OF THE BASIC STANCE—There are many variations to the basic stance mostly depending upon the position of the free foot. Have your model imagine two arcs, one small one, in which the free foot travels from the toe of the basic foot to the heel of the basic foot. The free foot can stop at any point within this arc—the toe (and the broad part of the kneecap) will always point in a line parallel to the camera-to-model line.

The large arc starts at a point beyond the toe with the leg of the free foot crossed over the basic foot/leg, and goes back to its own side beyond the heel of the basic foot with toe and broad part of the kneecap still pointing in a line parallel to the camera-model line.

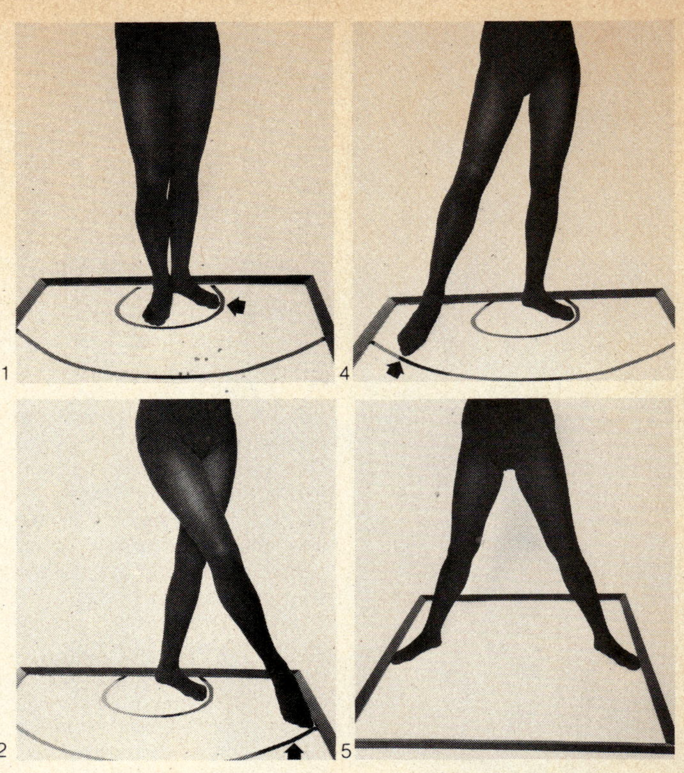

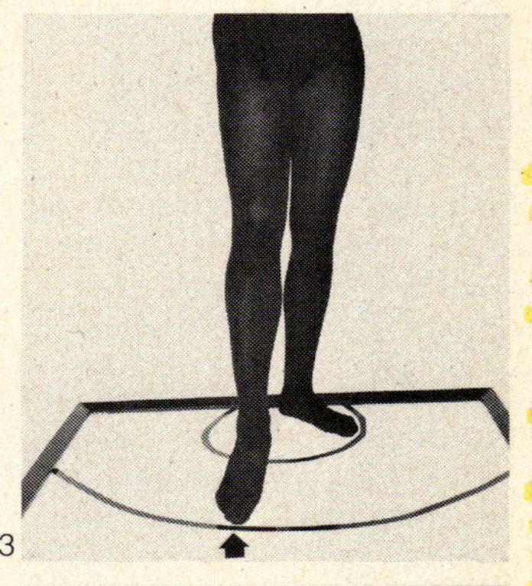

Lunge
Broken Zig Zag
Leg opposite tilt of head
Curved
Diagonal
Vertical

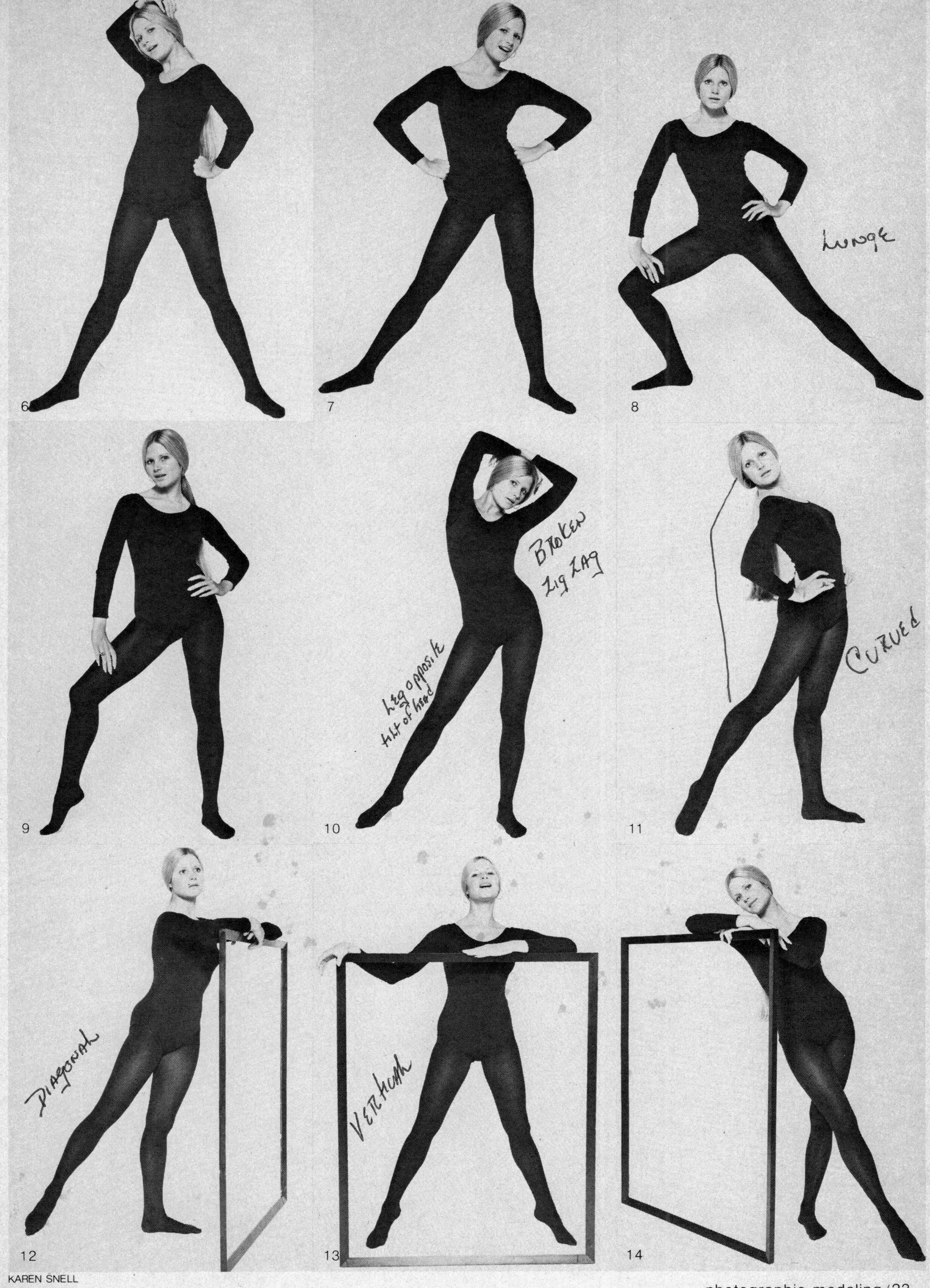

KAREN SNELL

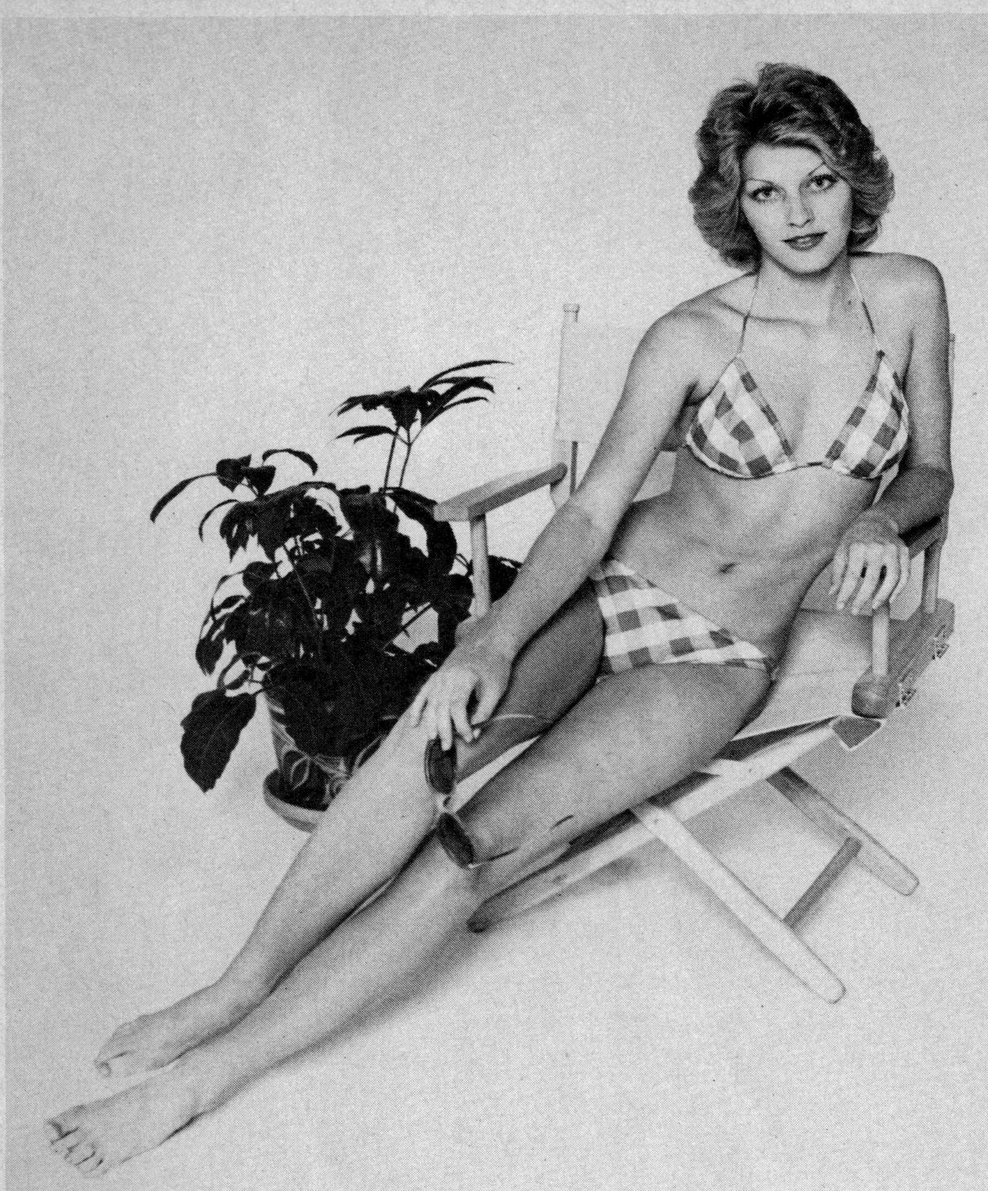

1

perhaps, a boyish look. One leg is kept straight with the toe on a diagonal line or pointing toward the camera while the other leg is bent at a sharp angle toward the side (as model is facing camera). The weight can be shifted to go onto the bent leg, requiring the model to angle her body toward the lunge, or the body can be held upright with the weight on the straight leg while the lunge effect is achieved by lifting the heel of the other foot.

BODY ANGLES

The basic positions a model assumes in photographic poses can be analyzed and separated into distinct categories. This analysis can prove to be very advantageous in helping a novice model gain knowlege of her body movements and, in so doing, help her develop versatility in movement. Standing positions can be separated into four categories: broken line, curved line, vertical and diagonal.

You and your model will need a straight edge of some kind and a few reference magazines to practice analyzing these body angles. Find full-length pictures with legs showing. Draw a line through the center of the model's head (even if the shot is a profile or ¾ picture, the line should be drawn through the center mass).

Connect the head line with a line drawn through the center of the body (an even amount of body shown on each side of the line). Now, draw a line from the lowest point of the torso line through the center of the free leg. (The supportive leg is the leg which holds the body's weight; the free leg bears no weight.)

THE BROKEN LINE—In a broken body line, the lines drawn through the head, body and leg create a zig-zag line, not continuous in a curved line or straight line. The head is tilted to the side, up or down in a reverse direction to the lines of the body. The leg goes

the lines of the garment are defined by the space between the legs and the contrast created by the costume and the background.

BASIC SPORTS STANCE— The model should stand with the legs apart, weight evenly distributed, toes pointing straight ahead or slightly outward.

VARIATIONS—The weight may be transferred to either leg, jutting the hip (corresponding to the weighted leg) out to the side. There are any number of variations that can be tried. For example: swing the hips and shoulders away from camera; swing hips away, leaving shoulders squared to camera, or swing shoulders away, leaving hips more or less facing the camera. The last alternative is generally limited to tall, thin models because this variation can be tricky and tends to make one seem short or hippy.

LUNGES—This stance is sometimes not suitable to soft, subtle fashions but is more likely to be used effectively with a garment that would be considered a strong fashion statement— ultrahigh fashion or,

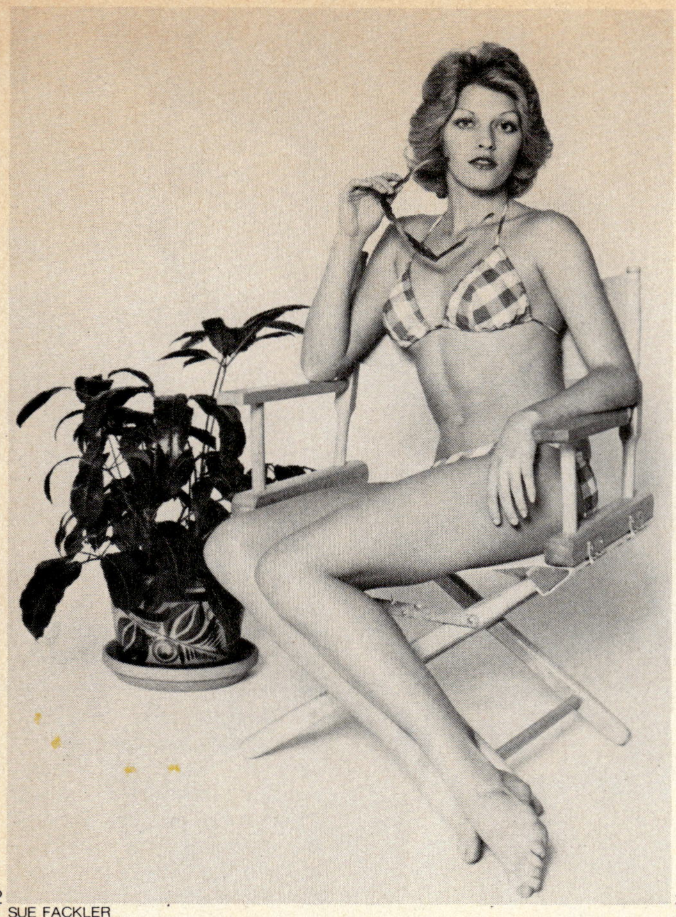

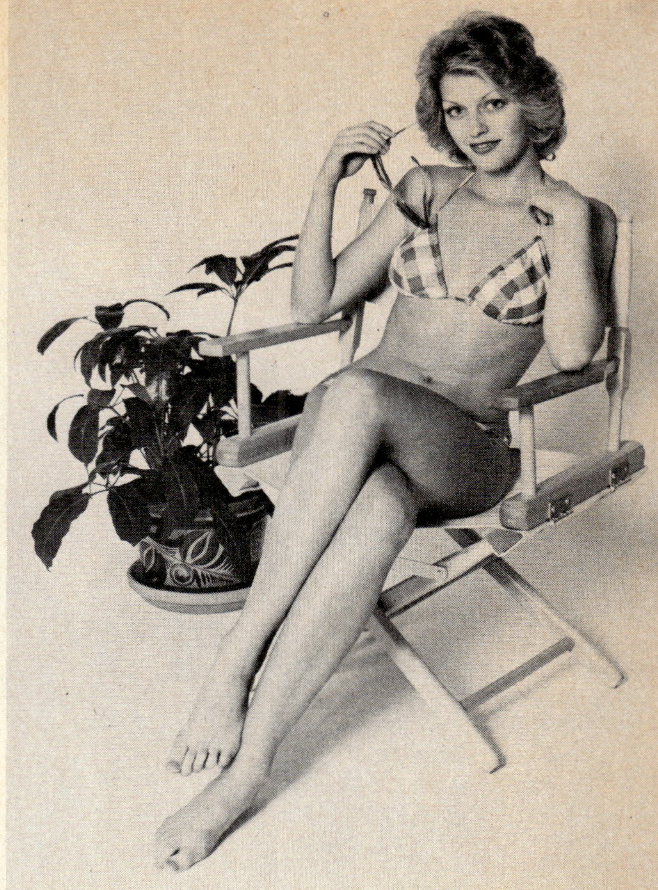

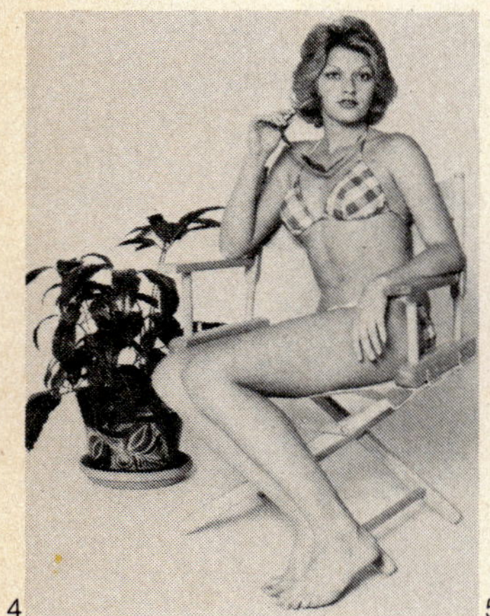

out at an angle opposite to the direction of the tilt of the head. This broken line is especially effective in creating fluid and mobile effects.

THE CURVED LINE—In the curved body line, the head is tilted to the side in a front shot, up or down in a profile shot, with the leg curved, bent or angled straight out in the same direction as the tilt of the head. The torso may or may not further accentuate the curve.

VERTICAL BODY LINES— The vertical line, although it may seem the simplest, is sometimes the most difficult body line to utilize and still achieve an effect of life and graceful lines in a picture. Much depends on facial expressions, arms and hands, subtle breaks in the leg or ankle line. You determine that a pose is based on a vertical line by drawing a line through the center of the head, body and through the free leg or between the legs if the weight is evenly distributed as in a sports stance.

DIAGONAL LINES—The body line is drawn through the face, torso and free leg to perform a perfect straight line at an angle to the floor. The body may be leaning backward against a railing or height for support with the free leg back to form a continuous diagonal line. The free leg might be crossed over going toward the back, or going forward

1. The obtuse sitting angle gives model a longer, frequently freer look, allows more of garment to be seen in fashion photographs.
2. 4. Feet should point same direction as knee-to-ankle line (2), or awkward pose results (4).
3. The right angle sitting position has line from neck through torso and line from hip bone through knee at 90-degree angle.
5. If legs are turned or curved toward outer ankle bone (foot turned inward), the foot looks uncontrolled or even broken.

to create a diagonal effect. A reasonable impression of balance must be created with use of arms or supportive props.

SITTING, RECLINING AND KNEELING POSES

Poses involving other than standing, walking, dancing and running situations can also be analyzed and understood by dividing them into three angular groups: right angle, obtuse angle and acute angle.

As in vertical poses, there are many factors to be considered in sitting, kneeling and reclining positions such as weight placement, flesh distortion, use of hands, legs or feet. To simplify the analysis so it can serve as a good foundation base of knowlege for these poses, the position of the head will not be considered in the following three angular analyses:

SITTING ANGLES—The sitting angle can be analyzed and determined by the line drawn from the neck through the mass of the torso, and from the hip bone to the knee bone (of the knee with the greater bend).

RIGHT ANGLE—The right angle sitting position might be created by a very prim pose with the knees together, sitting on the edge of a chair, or the feeling might swing all the way to the other side of the scale with a very geometric high fashion sprawl which specializes in a haughty disregard for grace and reaches out for a bony, angular feeling.

OBTUSE ANGLE—The obtuse-angled sitting position is generally more favored than the acute or right angle sitting positions in fashion shots since it allows more of

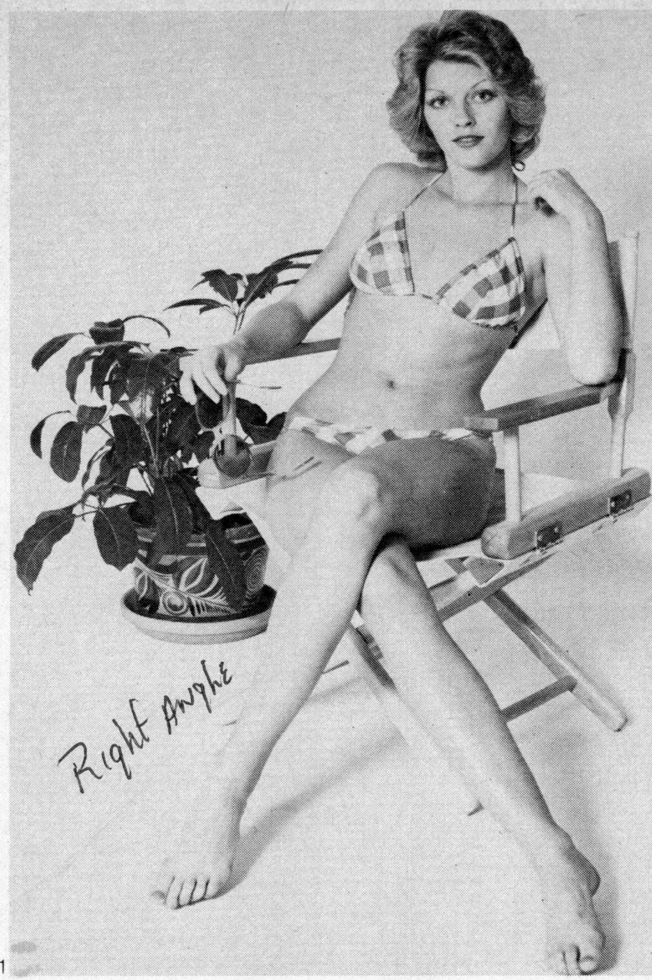

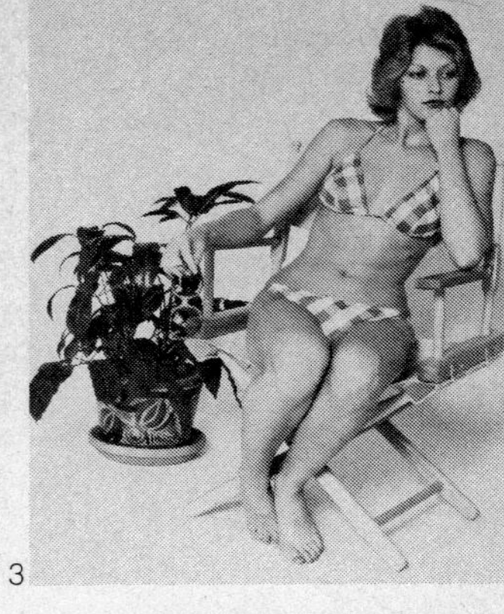

1. Legs should be crossed as high above the knee as possible to avoid flesh distortion.
2. Placing weight on hip away from camera results in heavy look to model's thigh.
3. Legs rarely look good tucked under the chair.
4. Model should remember to use spinal column for support.

the garment to be seen, and gives the model a longer, frequently freer, look. In this instance, when the lines are drawn from the neck through the torso and from the hip bone to the knee, the angle created is more than 90 degrees (or an obtuse angle).

ACUTE ANGLE—The torso line and the upper leg line form an acute angle or an angle less than 90 degrees in some sitting poses. Frequently, one leg is stretched out breaking the effect of the body being rolled up into a ball. Great care must be taken in these poses to avoid rolls of flesh or fabric in the midriff area.

HELPFUL HINTS IN SITTING POSES—Right angle sitting positions, especially, are

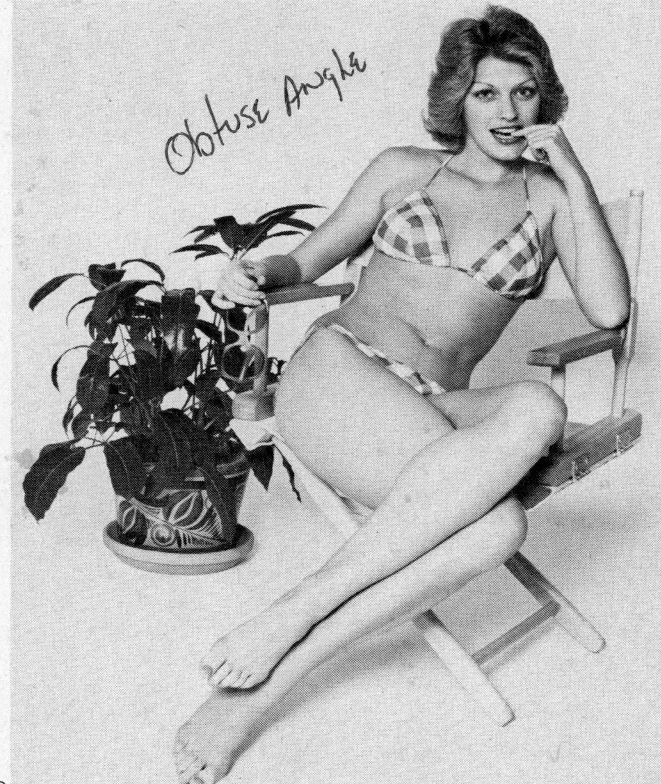

more flattering to the model when she places herself in a chair in such a manner that her upper leg line (from hips to knee) is in a diagonal line on the seat. Her lower leg should then be in a line going the opposite direction to balance the effect. An attractive zigzag composition will be the result.

Feet should always be pointing in the same direction as the knee-to-ankle line of the leg. When the line is reversed, an awkward impression results.

Ankles turned slightly in toward the inside of the ankle (foot turned outward) will give the leg a prettier line. If they are turned or curved toward the outer ankle bone (foot turned inward), the foot looks uncontrolled or even broken.

Legs rarely look their best when the model tucks them under the chair; it results in foreshortening, tenses the calf muscles and creates the illusion of fat legs.

Crossed legs should be crossed as high above the knee as possible to avoid flesh distortion. Be sure the bottom leg is out at least as far as (or under) the knee. The lower leg (from knee to ankle) may fall parallel, or top leg dropped straight from the knee to the floor with the under-leg (with toes pointed) angled out to the side.

Obtuse-angled sitting poses generally require the model to place her weight on one buttock or the other (exception, sitting flat on the backside, leaning back on arms). If showing fashion is the motivation of the photograph, the model will show more of the garment if she rests her weight on the hip closer to the camera. The smooth, unflattened curve of the hipline created by placing the weight on the hip furthest from the camera is frequently desirable for glamour shots.

The model should always remember to utilize her spinal column for support even when seemingly leaning on an arm or elbow. Distortions of shoulder sockets and elbows should be avoided.

Sitting positions cause extra wrinkling in clothes and rolls in the flesh when

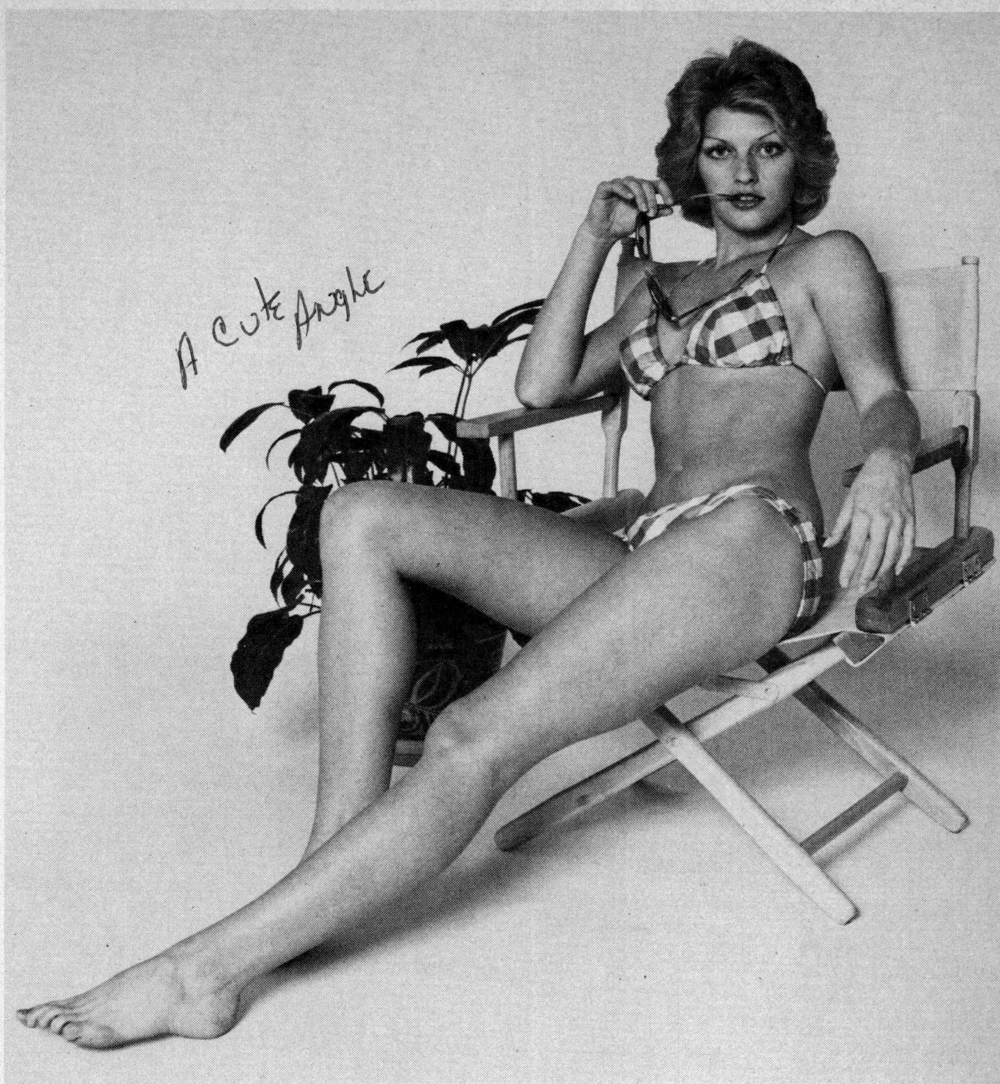

exposed. Care should be taken to maintain as much smoothness as possible around the waistline.

KNEELING POSES—Kneeling positions are generally right angled or acute (determination of the angle is torso to knees, and knees to ankle), on the weighted leg or legs. Variations in kneeling positions may be created by kneeling on one knee only and placing the other leg in front with the foot placed flat on the floor.

Knee of the unweighted leg will be bent at a right angle or in a semistraightened, or straightened position.

As in standing poses the free leg is then free to travel in an arc—starting with the knee and foot crossed over

the body, and moving clear over to the other side stopping any point on the arc. Many interesting effects can be achieved by stopping the foot on different points of the arc.

As in the standing position, the free foot should generally point toward the camera lens except in a lungelike effect where deliberate angularity in effect is desired.

Additional variations in the free-leg/weighted-leg kneeling position can be created by adjusting the height of the knee by bringing it toward the center

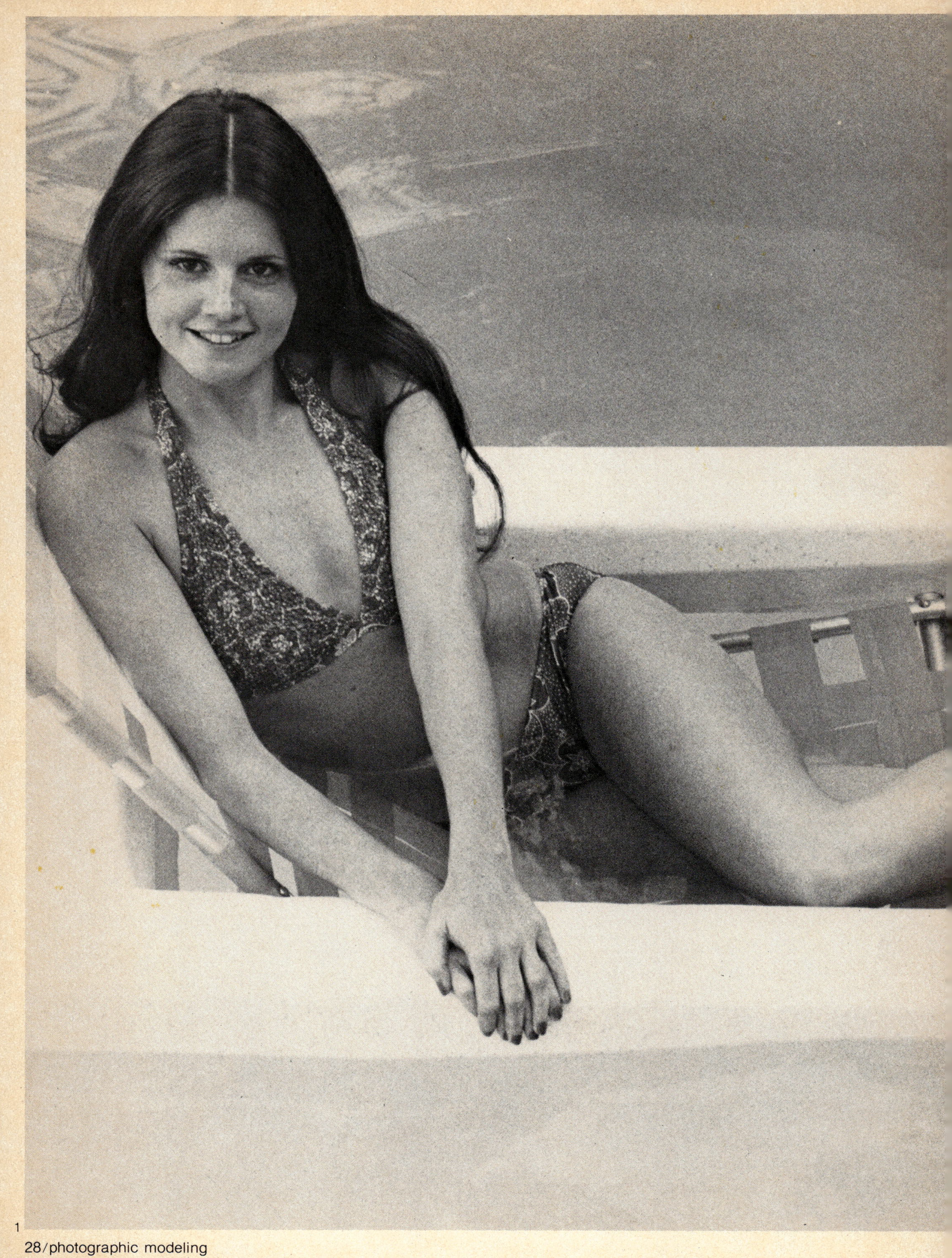

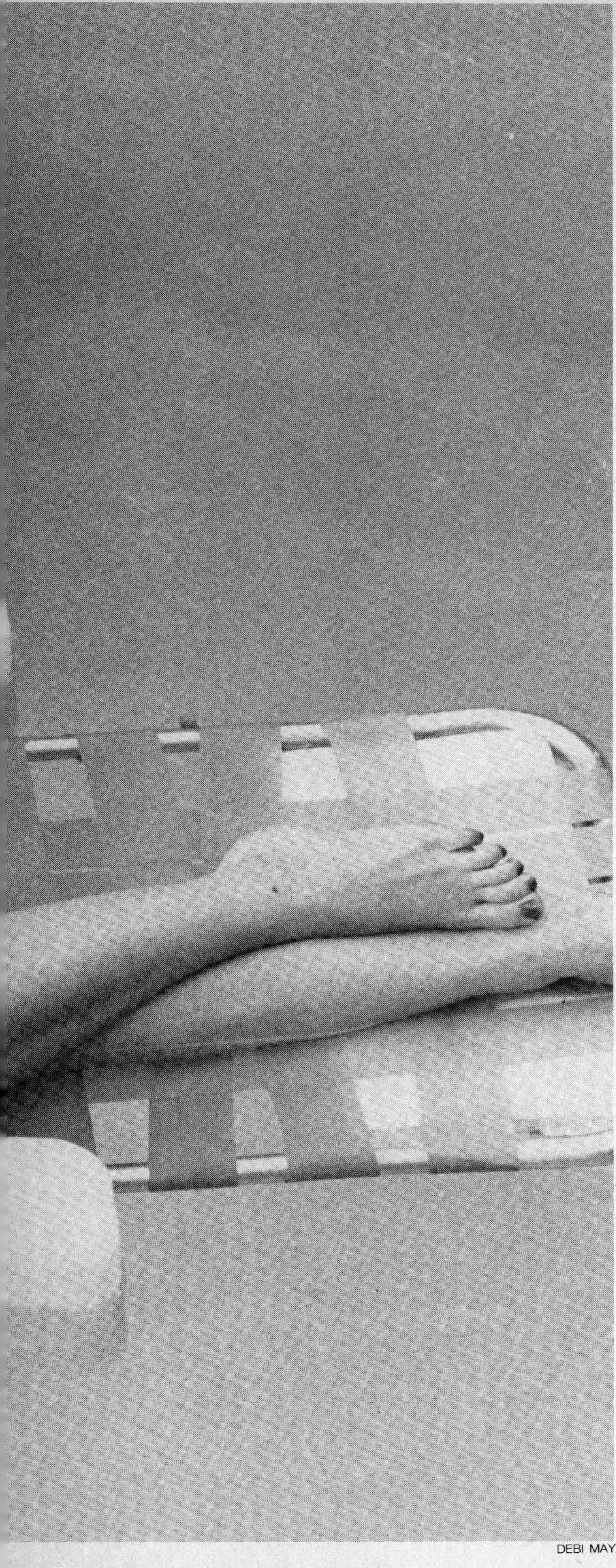

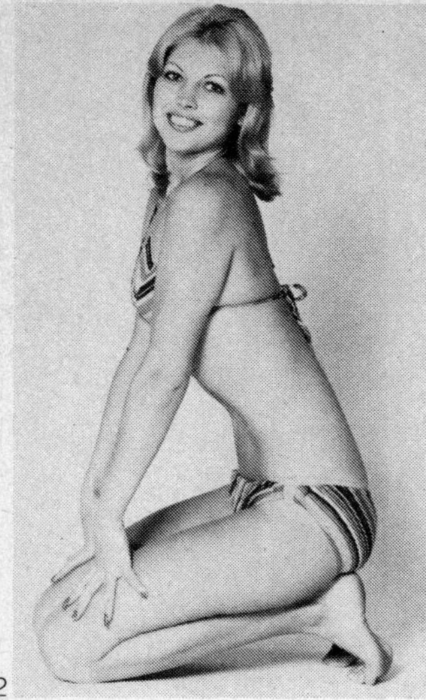

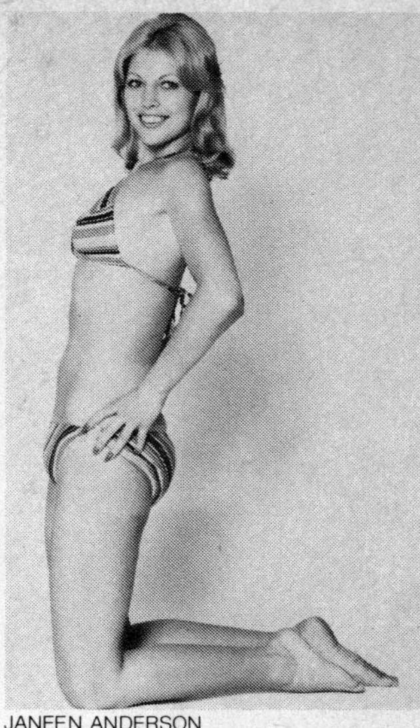

2

3

JANEEN ANDERSON

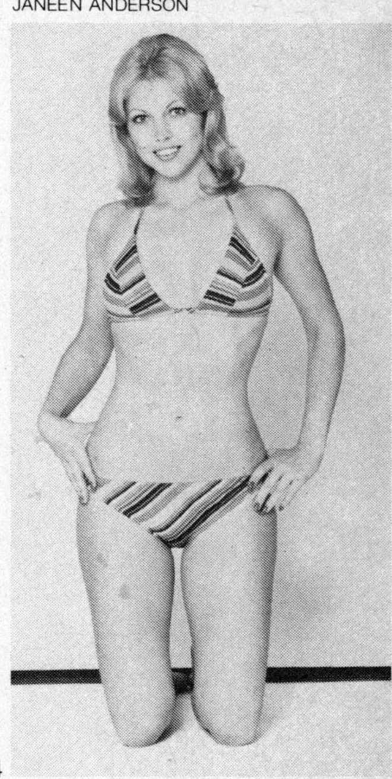

4

of the body line and lowering the knee toward the floor. As in standing poses, the model's body may be positioned to face the camera, have one side to the camera or with the back to the camera—or any point in between the full 360-degree circle.

HELPFUL HINTS IN KNEELING POSES—The photographer should understand that kneeling on a hard surface for any length of time can be not only uncomfortable, but actually very painful. He should avoid asking the model to maintain an uncomfortable position beyond a reasonable few minutes.

Unfortunate optical illusions might be created if the calf and foot of at least one of the model's legs (preferably both) is not at least partially exposed to camera view. If the lower part of the leg is not at least indicated, it could easily look like you're model had lost her lower legs.

1. In reclining poses, body should be supported by spinal column as much as possible so that weight on supporting arm(s) won't cause shoulder to look disjointed and unattractive.
2. Kneeling positions are classified depending on angle between torso and knees, and between knees and ankles.
3. Soles of feet are not photo- genic. Encourage model to alter pose to avoid showing them.
4. Calf and foot of at least one leg should be at least partly exposed to camera or it could look like model has lost her lower legs.

DEBI MAY

The soles of the feet (and often soles of shoes) are not especially photogenic. Encourage the model to alter her pose to avoid photographing this area.

RECLINING POSITIONS—A model may place herself in a reclining or semireclining position, on her side, her back or her stomach. If the purpose is to show as much of the garment as possible, the model should rest on her side and turn the body toward the camera. She might want to bend one knee slightly and perhaps steady herself with the unweighted hand for balance. It is generally less complicated if the model bends her top leg—and lovely hipline and leg curves can be achieved without losing sight of the other leg or a portion thereof.

It is important, in many cases for the model to support herself with her elbow or elbows so she can manage to make her face more visible to the camera. In these cases, it is important for the body to be supported by the spinal column as much as possible and as little weight as is absolutely necessary is transferred to the arm. If all the weight is on the supporting arm or arms, the shoulder might appear disjointed and unattractive. If the camera is above the model reclining on her back, her poses will require a little twisting and turning to break up the body line and lend interest to the pose and pictorial composition.

On the preceding pages the analysis of standing, sitting and kneeling poses was mostly addressed to

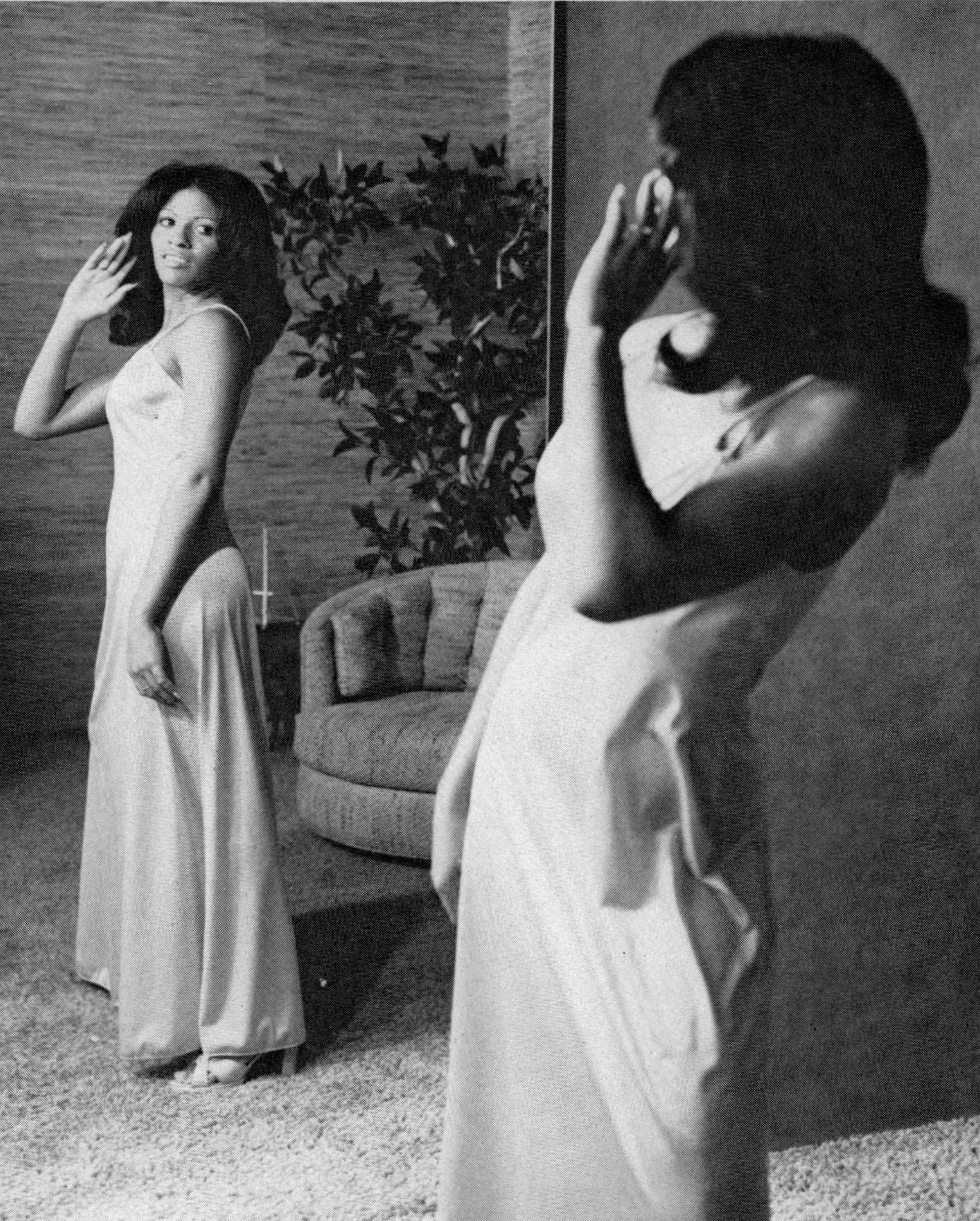

vertical lines and their variations (curved, broken or zig-zag lines, straight, diagonal).

Increased mobility in posing and interest in body angles can be achieved by utilizing horizontal lines and varying their relation to each other and to the vertical lines.

To simplify understanding of these all-important elements in posing, the model in the accompanying photographs is wearing transparent blocks—the upper one indicating the

chest block and the lower one indicating the hip block. The hip block is marked with an X to indicated the weighted hip (the hip which corresponds to the leg upon which the model is standing).

The hip and chest block variations are easy to understand and, when used

Model should practice stances in front of mirror to see just what they look like.

along with the basic vertical body angle information, one becomes aware of the infinite number of poses and positions possible. Lines at either side of the model represent the lines perpendicular to the floor or vertical line. □

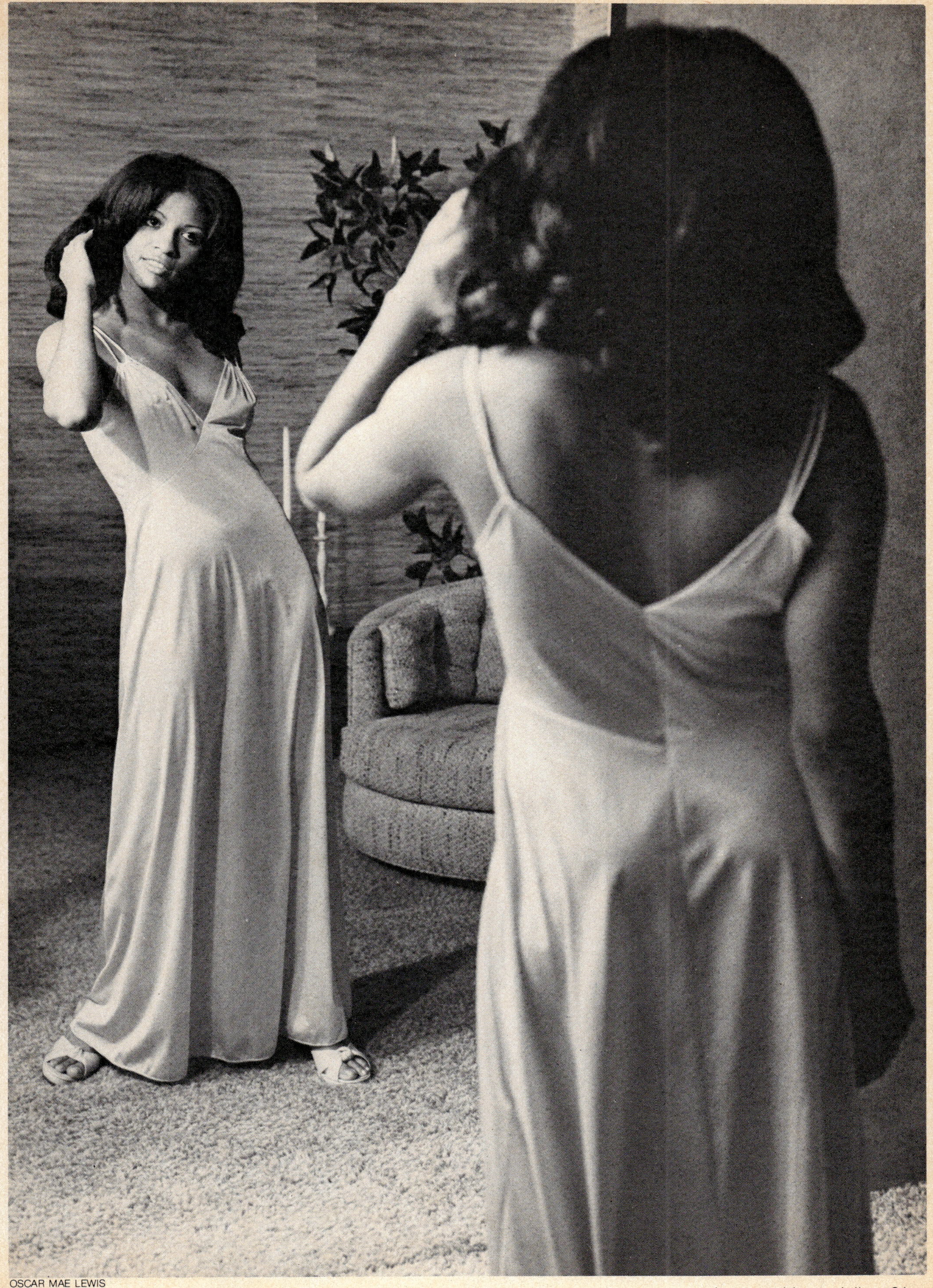

OSCAR MAE LEWIS

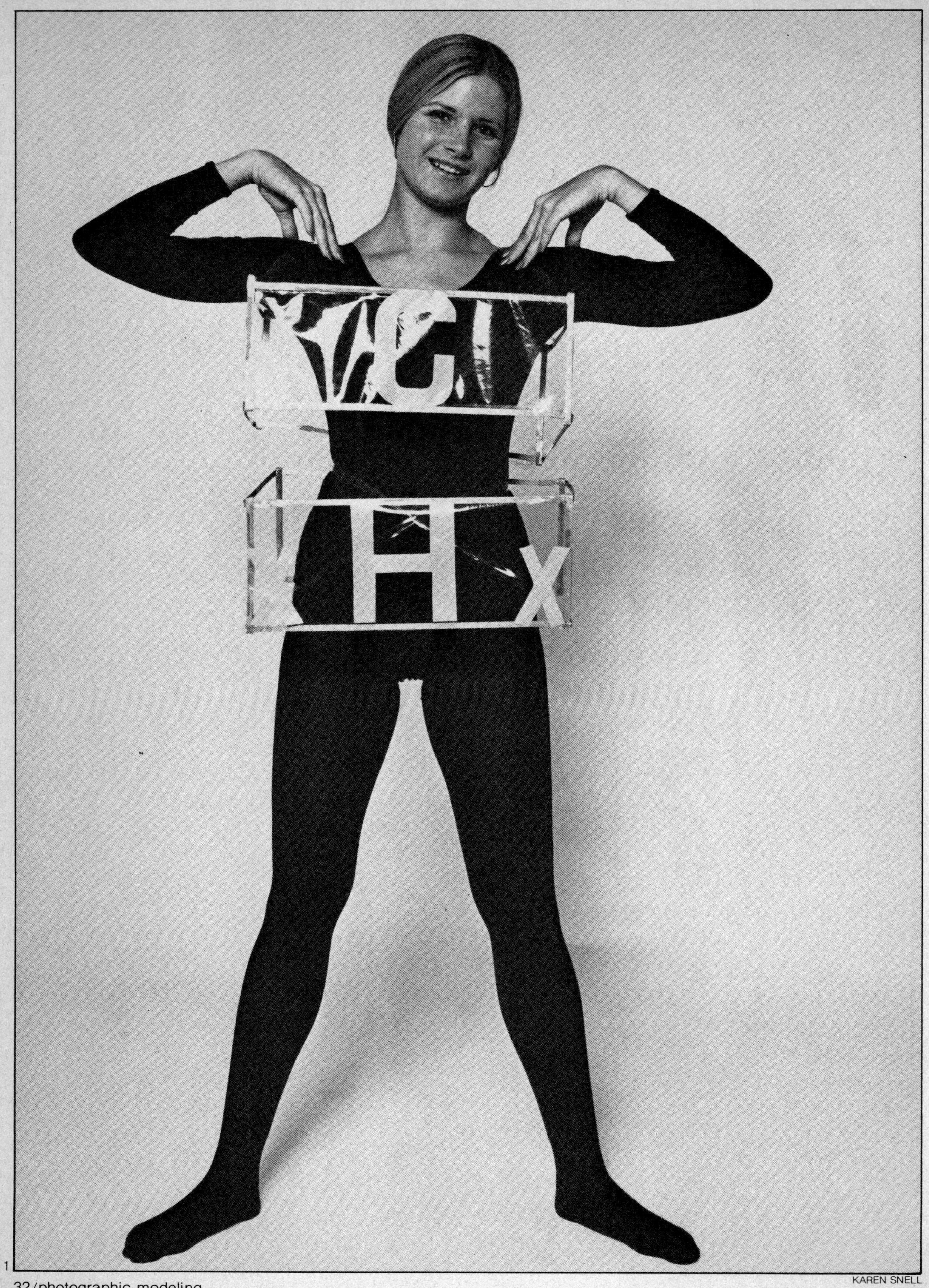

KAREN SNELL

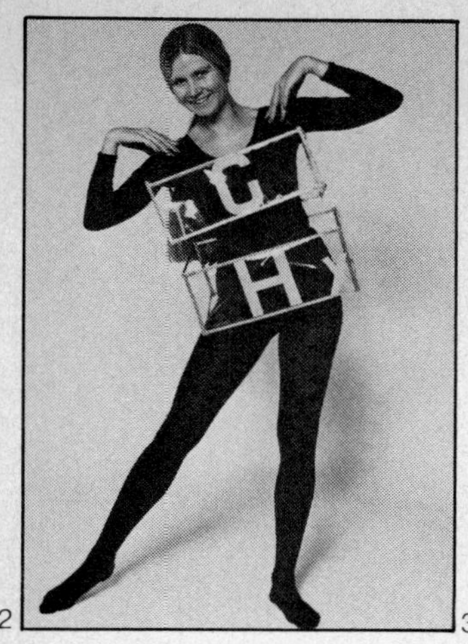
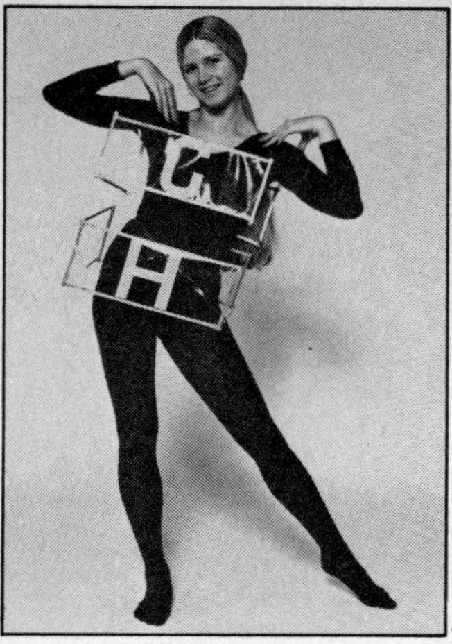
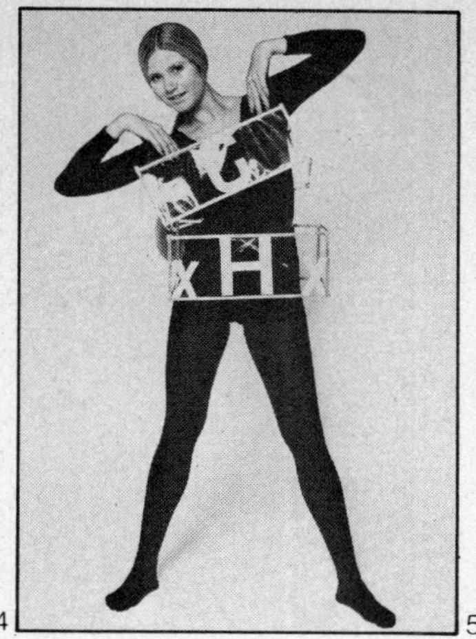
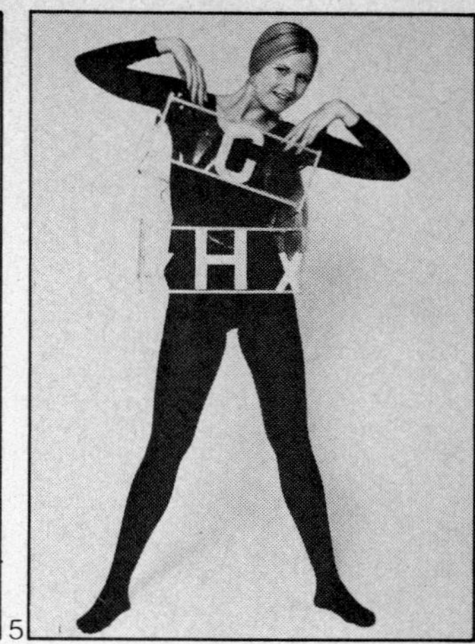
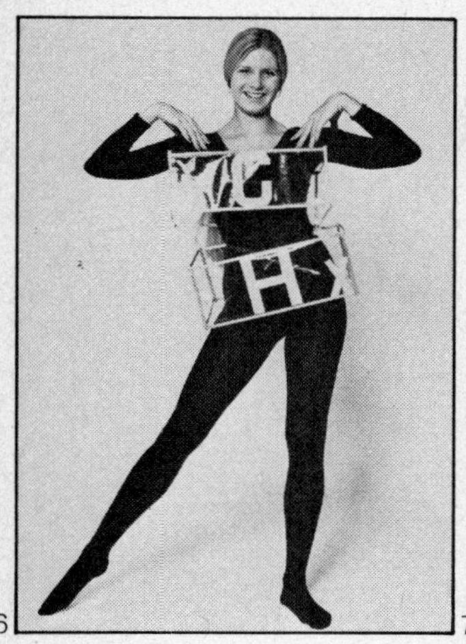
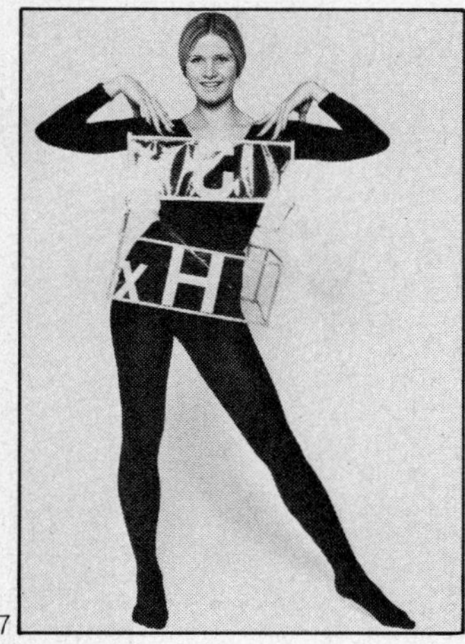
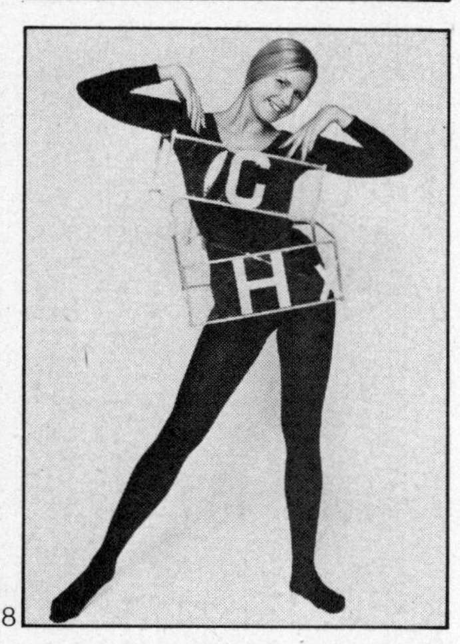

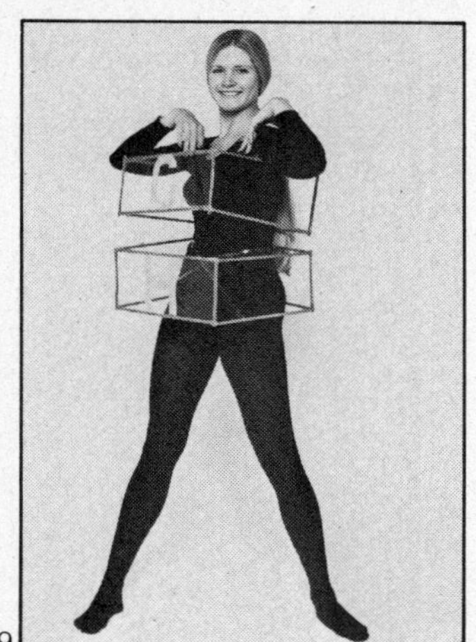

1. Chest and hips parallel and level. Weight is evenly distributed here between legs.
2. Chest and hips parallel and tilted down to right. Weight is on left leg.
3. Chest and hips parallel and tilted down to left. Weight is on right leg.
4. Chest tilted down to right and hips level. Weight is evenly distributed on both legs.
5. Chest tilted down to left and hips level. Weight is evenly distributed on both legs.
6. Chest level and hips tilted down to right. Weight is on the model's left leg.
7. Chest level and hips tilted down to left. Weight is on the model's right leg.
8. Chest tilted to left and hips tilted to right. Weight is on the model's left leg.
9. Chest twisted to right and hips twisted to right.

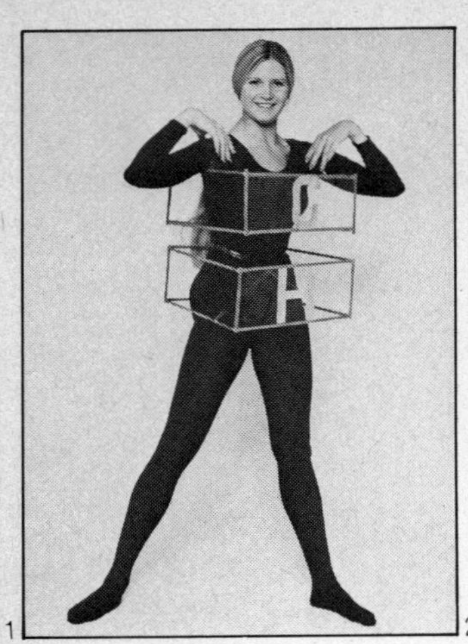 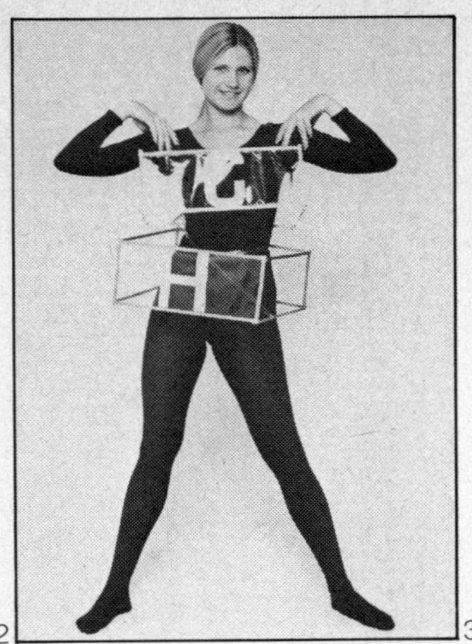 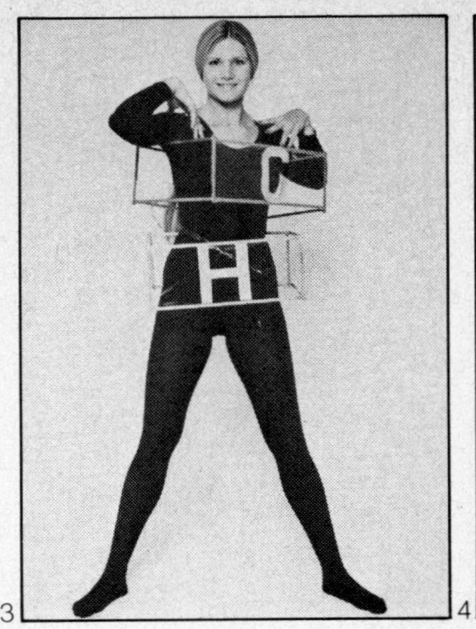 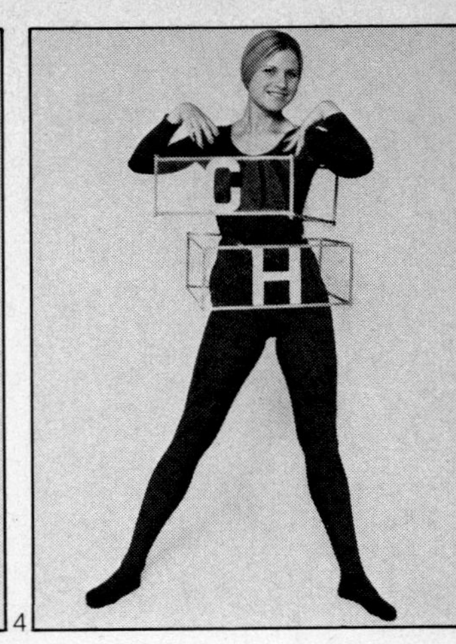

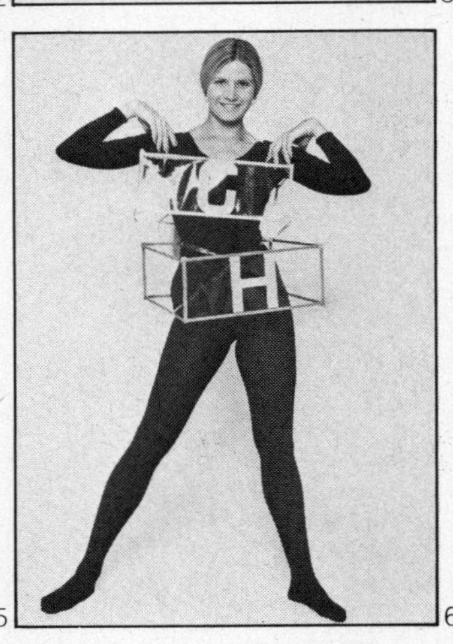 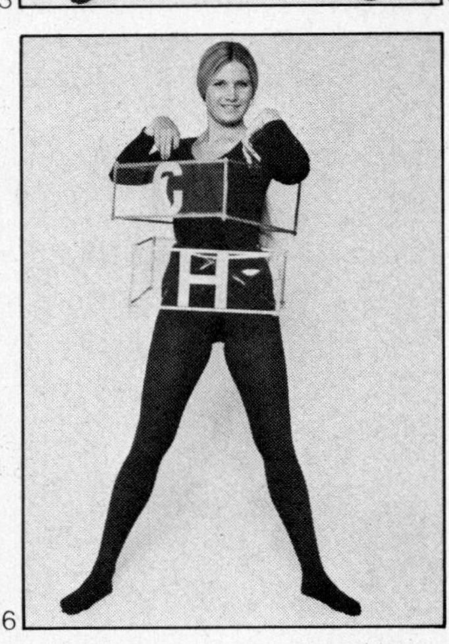

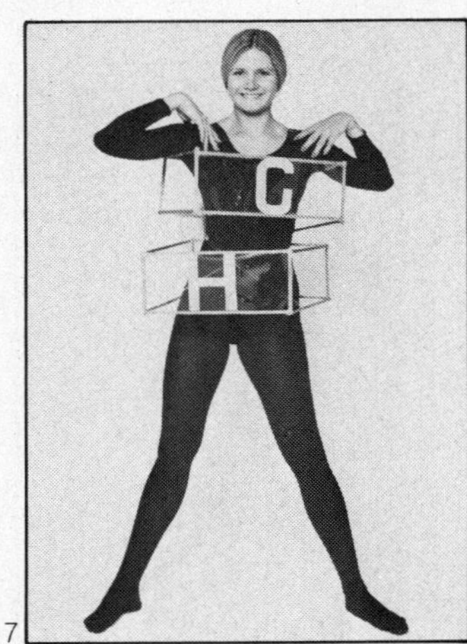

1. Chest twisted to left and hips twisted to left.
2. Chest facing camera and hips twisted to right.
3. Chest twisted to left and hips facing camera.
4. Chest twisted to right and hips twisted to left.
5. Chest facing camera and hips twisted to left.
6. Chest twisted to right and hips facing camera.
7. Chest twisted to left and hips twisted to right.
8. Combination: Chest twisted to right and hips twisted to left and tilted to left. All twist and tilt combinations will work and should be practiced often in front of a mirror.

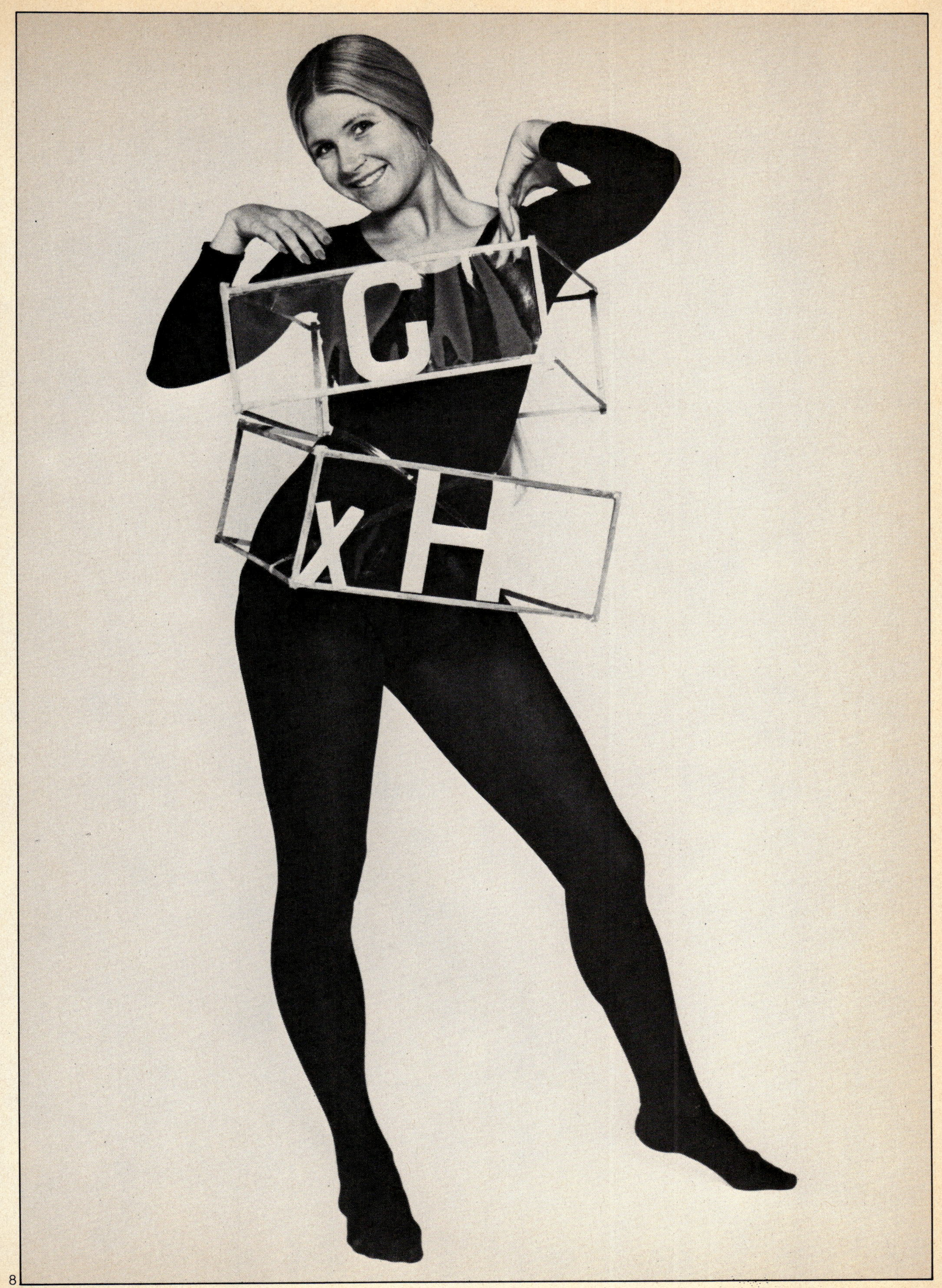
C
x H

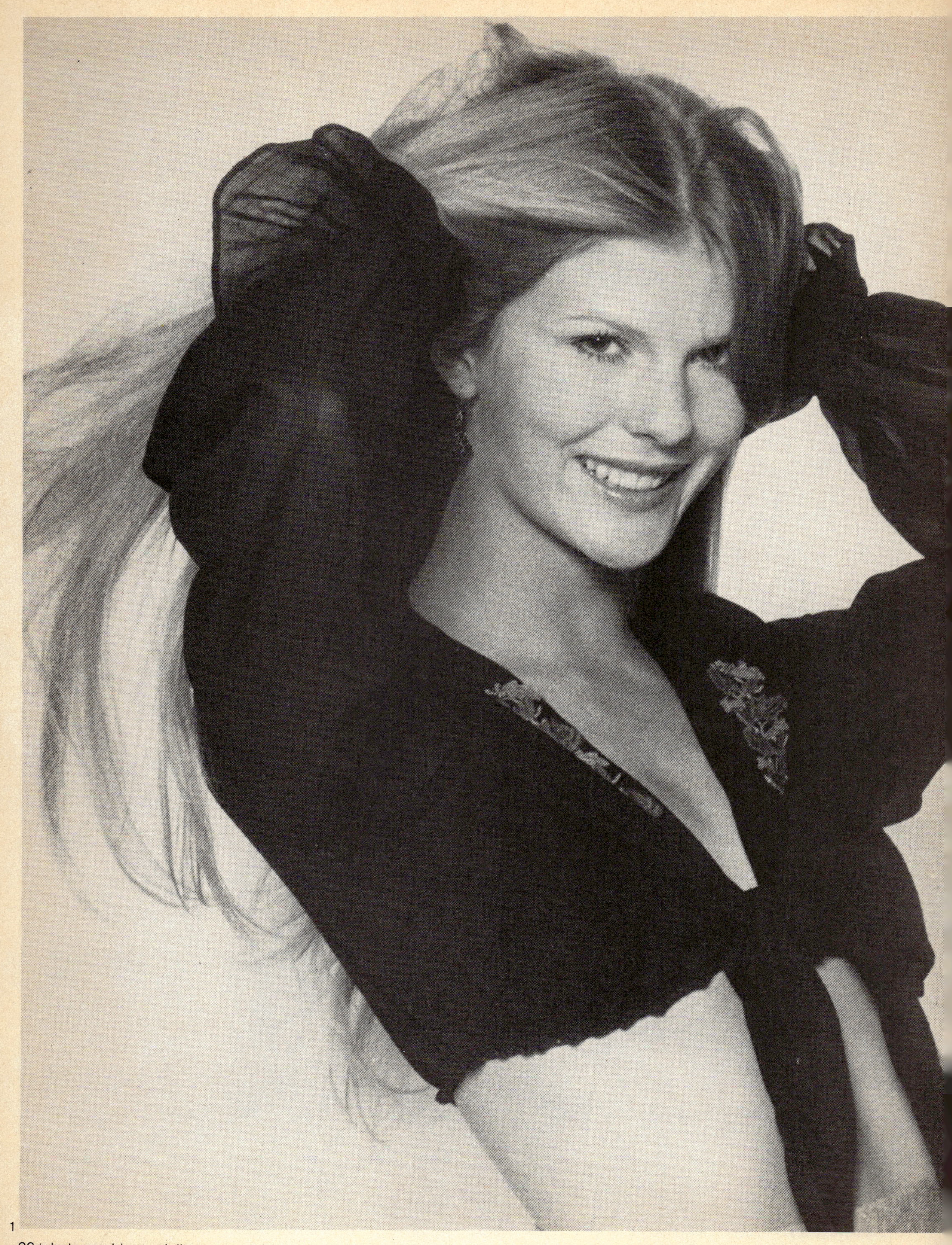

relations, or other commercial areas that employ photo graphics).

The reason? First of all, if a photo editor considers you an important photography resource, he or she is not going to jeopardize your working relationship. If he or she doesn't consider you an important photography resource, then, in the photo editor's mind your photography probably isn't worth stealing.

Secondly, the publishers you contact, should be the familiar ones. Check a PHOTOGRAPHER'S MARKET of three years ago to see which publishers are in the present (1981) PHOTOGRAPHER'S MARKET. Finally, most houses you will be dealing with through a directory such as PHOTOGRAPHER'S MARKET or a market letter such as THE PHOTOLETTER are large -- anywhere

continued on page 4

Coming...

Annual Marketing Issue
Starting your own business
More portraiture, Creative
 Edge, Art of Seeing
Big API contest

IS THIS YOUR LAST ISSUE?

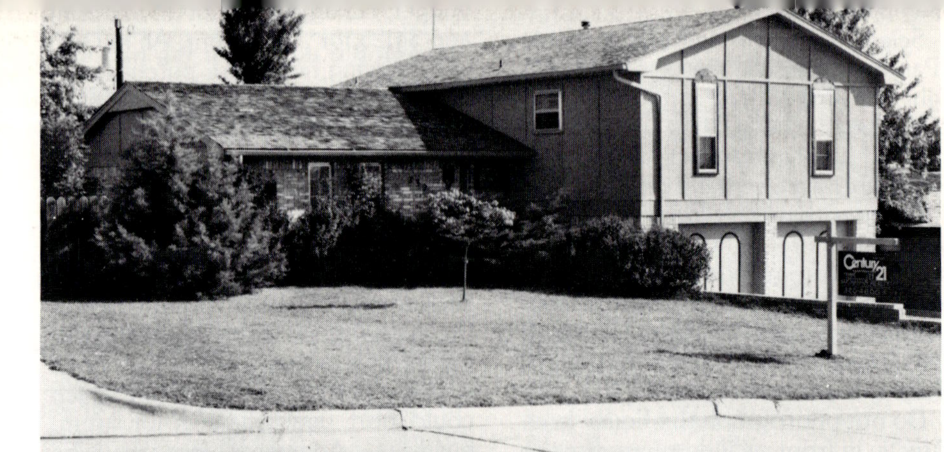

The real estate market is booming and looks like it will never quit. While others are making fortunes, large and small, you can get a chunk of the pie for yourself.
This article, and others, provide some great ideas on how you can get your share.

Before approaching a realtor with your ideas, go out and photograph several houses in your area, for sale or not, to use as samples of your work. Choose a home with a minimum of clutter in the yard, such as children's toys or automobiles. Print 5"x7" B/W photographs just as you would if you were doing them for a client.

For exposure, follow this simple rule: expose for the shadows, develop for the highlights. In order to do this, take an exposure reading of the shadows then of the highlighted areas. Average these two readings favoring the shadow exposure. For example, if your reading for the shadow is f4 and for the highlighted areas f11, set the exposure at about f5.6. When developing your film, underdevelop slightly (10-20%). This will give good shadow detail, while not allowing the brightly lighted areas to "block-up." The reason I recommend this technique is that many newpapers are

continued on page 2

Associated Photographers International

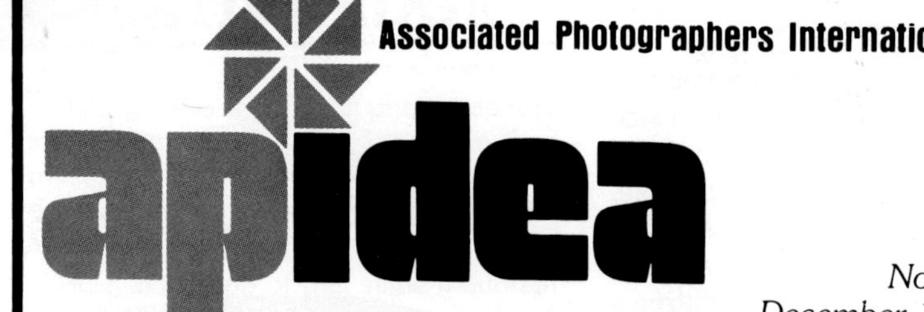

No. 90
December 1980

Serving a network of 18.000 Freelance Photographers throughout the U S
and in 105 countries sharing money-making and money-saving ideas!

Return Postage Guaranteed
21822 Sherman Way
Canoga Park, CA 91303

THERE'S MONEY IN REAL ESTATE PHOTOS

A "Land Office" Business

by Tim S. Hallen, Norman, OK © 1980

Few people realize the potential part-time earnings available in real estate photography. Just a quick glance through the newspaper will reveal many possible markets.

Many realtors take their own photographs using inexpensive "instant" cameras in order to keep their expenses down. They seldom realize that the less-than-adequate quality of these photographs may hinder the quick sale of a home. A few extra dollars spent by them with a good freelancer (YOU!) will actually **increase** their sales potential.

SPECIAL EXCLUSIVE REPORT TO API

Hot Markets

by Rohn Engh,
Publisher "The Photoletter"

Pirating Your Pictures

What about **piracy?** Could a photo editor use your picture and not pay for it? Contrary to the fiction you may have read elsewhere, such piracy rarely exists in the photo illustration field (we cannot speak for the field of advertising, public

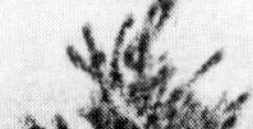

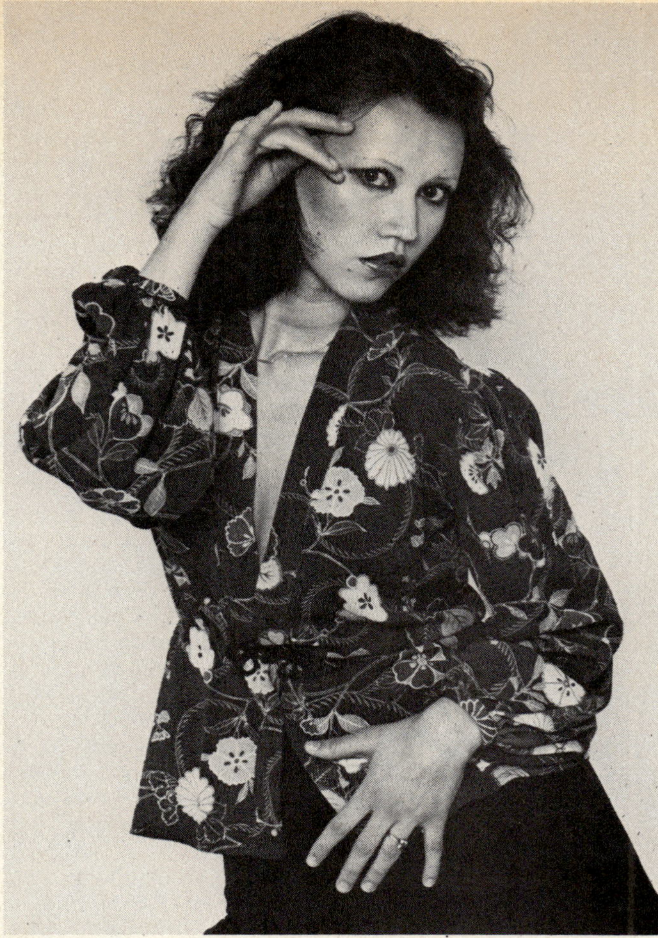

2

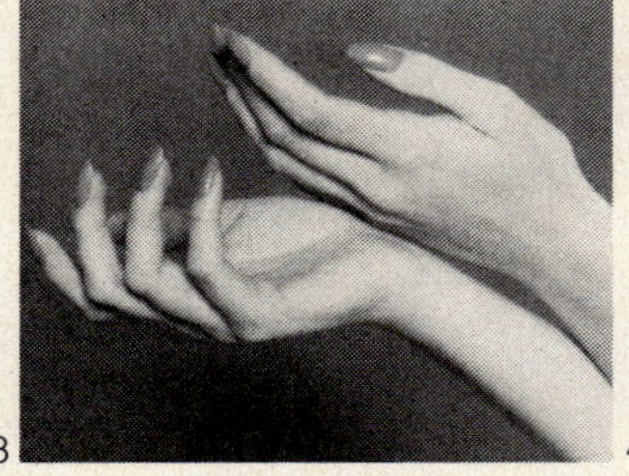

3

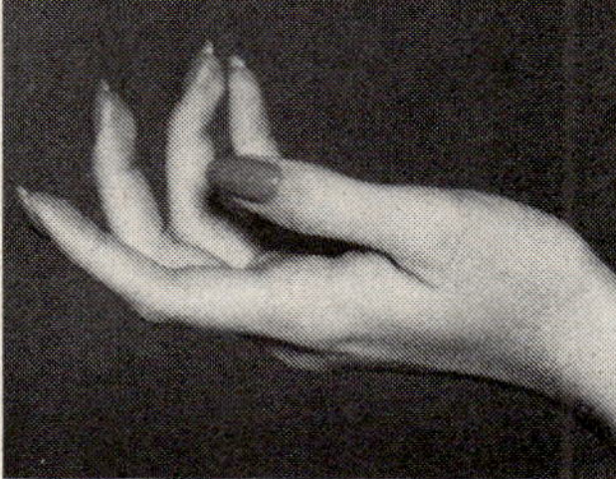

4

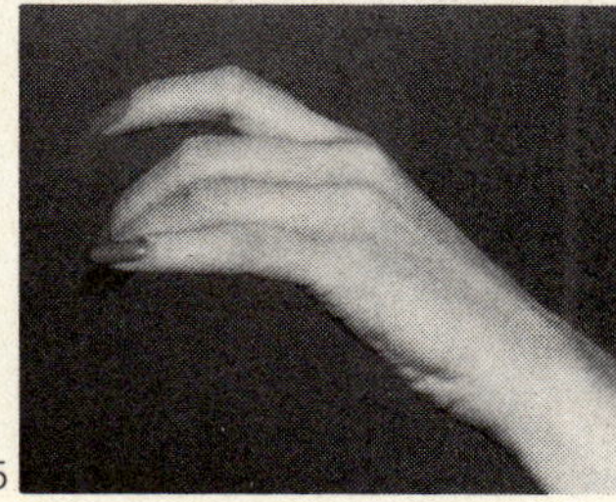

5

1, 2. Running the hands through the hair is a natural gesture. The variations of these movements are as infinite as the moods that inspire them.
3. Generally, the hands are turned so that the profile or semiprofile is visible to the camera or viewer.
4. Tapering the fingers so that the little finger is curved in toward the palm and the index finger is nearly straight produces graceful effect.
5. Alternative graceful finger arrangement is with third and fourth fingers together and bent slightly toward palm.

THE HANDS

The model's hands are used to create a mood, to call attention to a particular feature of a garment or to utilize or display a prop.

The best photographic gestures are done with a rather light touch. From time to time, a strong, heavy technique might be used for sportswear or some special effect, but ordinarily a model should think of her arms as being weightless.

Generally, the hands are turned so that the profile, or a semiprofile is visible to the camera. In other words, the hand is turned sideways so that the thumb side or the little finger side is turned closer to the camera.

The full front or back of the hand would usually be shown only for special effects, especially for gloves, jewelry, fingernail or cosmetic shots. With the exception of these specific shots the fingers should not be held tightly together or spread out.

More graceful effects can be created by tapering the fingers so that the little finger is curved in toward the palm and the index finger is nearly straight. A stiff, pointing effect of the index finger should be avoided.

An alternate graceful finger arrangement is with the third and fourth fingers together and bent slightly toward the palm. (Index and little finger are less pointed.)

The naturally talented model will instinctively follow through with any mood with appropriate hand gestures. When she is trying to be sporty, she will automatically create a fist and place them on her hips, hook her thumbs in suspenders or in the waistline of her pants or

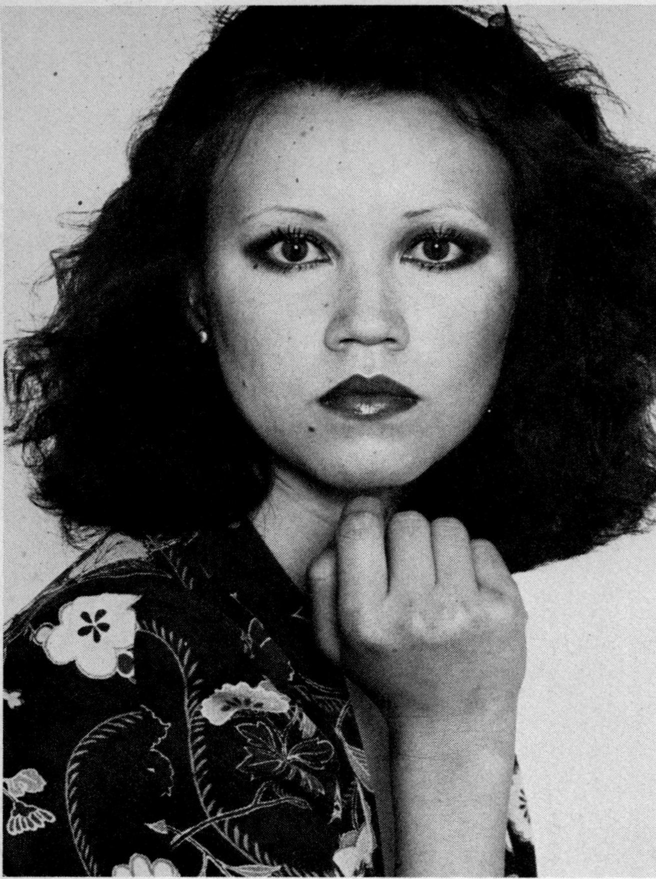

NANCY MANNFOLK

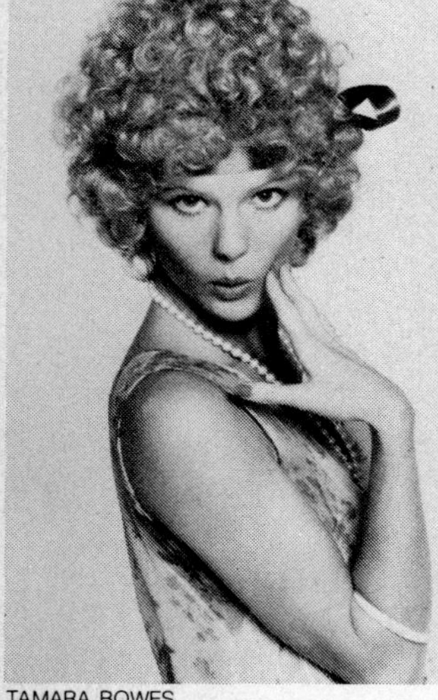

TAMARA BOWES

Women and girls frequently touch their faces as natural reaction to their many emotions, and this represents a good use of hands for photos.

the moods which inspire them. It might be a lioness running all her fingers through her hair in a strongly seductive movement; a shy, sweet young thing just barely touching her hair, or an outdoor girl feeling very alive using the same gesture as the lioness in a different context to express her freedom.

HANDS AND FACE—Women and girls quite frequently touch their faces as a natural reaction to their many emotions. A model might bring her hand to her mouth and just touch or bite her thumb or any one of her fingers. She might rest her chin on a fist or the open palm, the back of her hand or she might touch her cheek with her fingers or place the entire palm against it. She might smooth her forehead or brow with a couple of fingers, shade her eyes or cover her mouth as if to express surprise or conceal a giggle. Point out to your model as many examples as you can find of models touching their faces—it will open up limitless posing possibilities for you, too.

A word of caution: Remember to instruct the model not to distort the flesh when she touches her face with her hands. The hands should barely touch with no excess pressure which may push or pull the flesh.

The model's first experiments in touching the face and hair are her first steps in learning to establish a mood with the help of her hands.

skirt, or do something equally pert and sassy—almost without thinking.

More graceful garments should inspire prettier hand movements. There are, however, ways of helping the model who does not naturally use her hands well to become more expressive and graceful in her hand movements.

Have your model sit in front of the mirror and practice pretty hand positions while she works on her facial expressions. Touching the face or hair comes naturally to women—once a model learns to utilize her hands as well as her face to express an emotion she is feeling, gestures in full length shots will come easier to her.

HANDS OR FINGERS— Running the hands through the hair is a natural feminine and expressive gesture. The variations of these movements are as infinite as

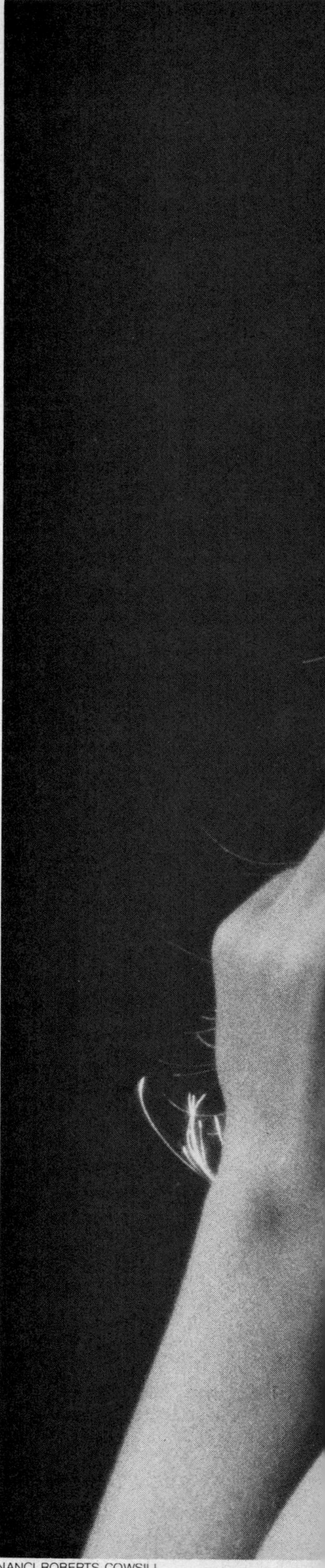

NANCI ROBERTS COWSILL

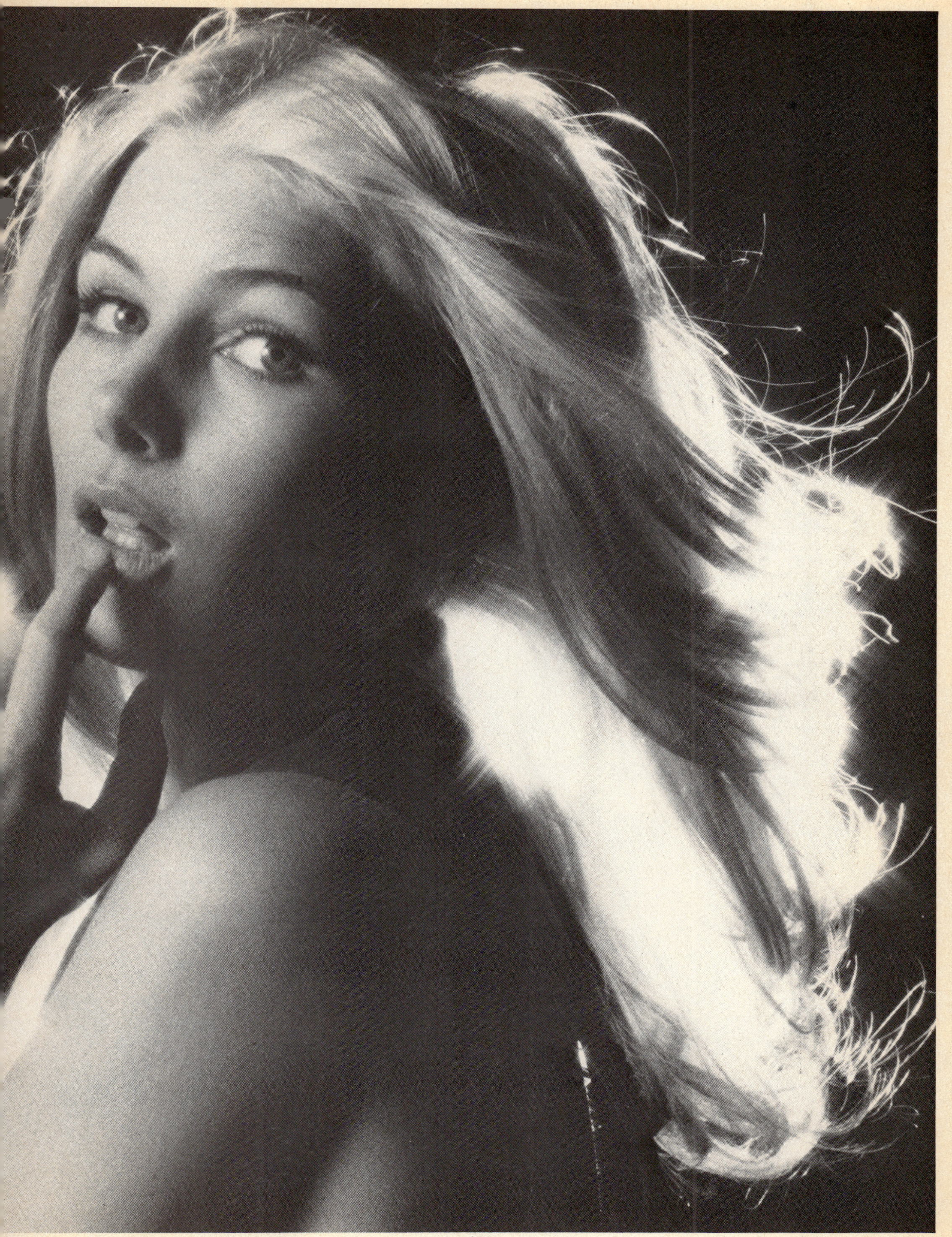

Each garment and each photographic situation provides a challenge to the model in expressing a mood. She must learn to relate to the feeling of the garment and scene and then relay a message through the poses she assumes.

Although the model must be encouraged to use her own natural gestures, there are some very basic hand positions frequently used by models that can provide a foundation for the wider variety of personal movements.

FINGERTIPS OR HANDS ON THIGHS—A good model standby is the placement of the fingertips or hands on the thighs. One of the reasons that this is a popular pose (especially in catalogue and merchandising shots) is that it makes it possible to show the entire garment without concealing any line or detail with the arms and hands. Also, the soft curve of the arm is generally more desirable than a sharp angle or bend.

There are four basic variations of the hand and finger placement on the thighs: The tips of the third finger or the thumb just barely touching the thigh, back of wrist gently curved outward; the entire palm of the hand and fingers placed on the thigh; the heel of the hand placed on the hip with the inside of the wrist turned in and fingers in a clenched or semiclenched position; and full fingers against hips with the palm of the hand curved away from the hip.

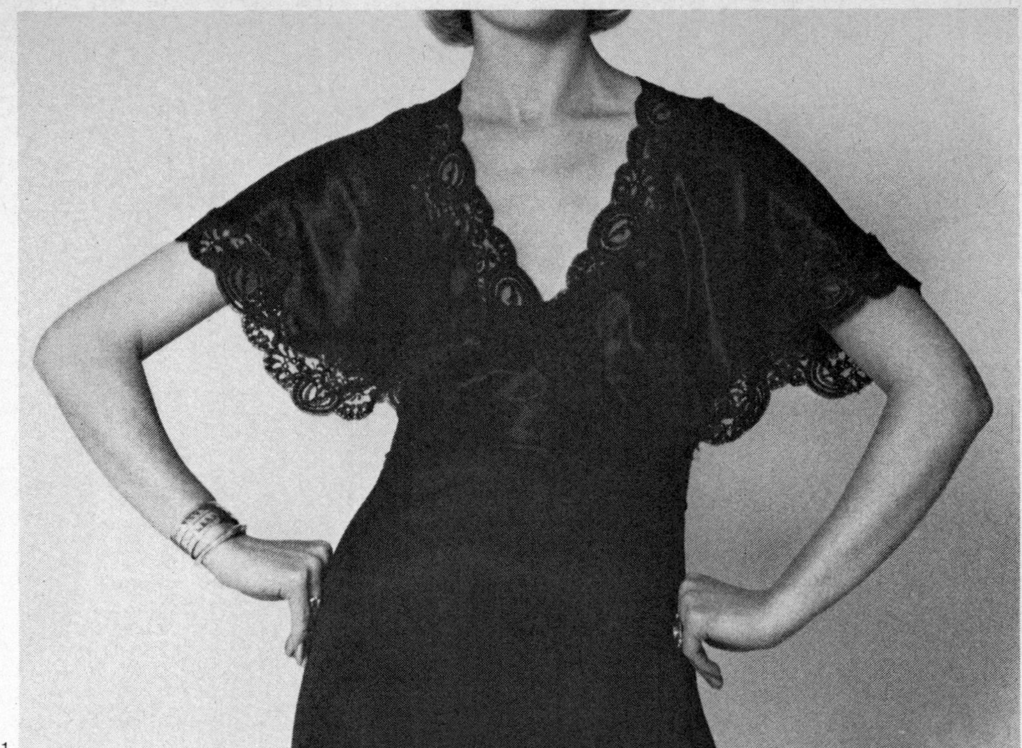

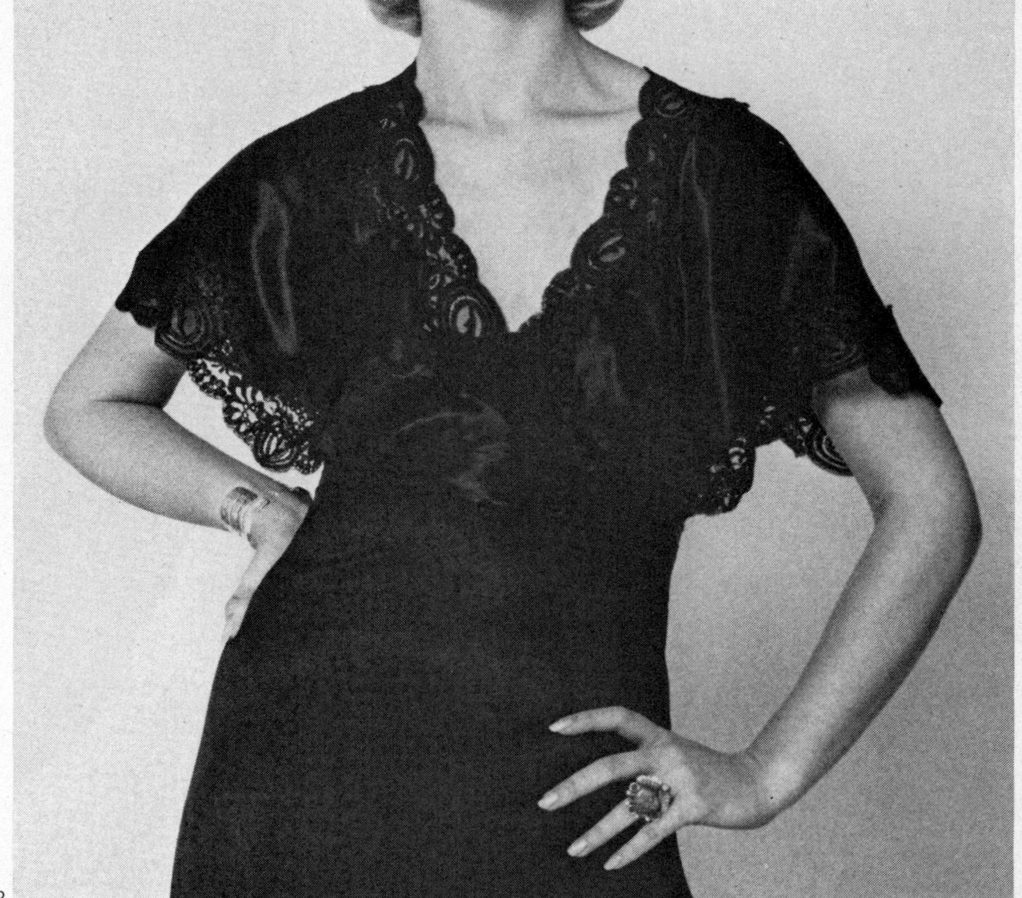

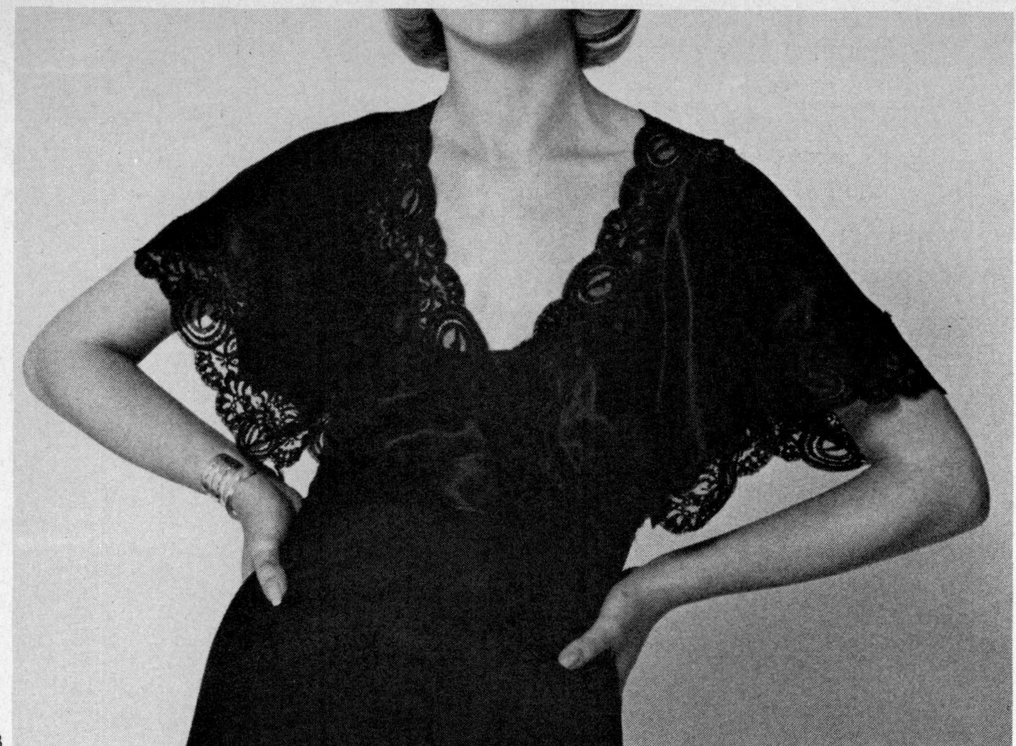

HANDS ON WAIST—When the fashion defines the natural waistline, it is quite suitable and often desirable to place the hands on the waist for emphasis and to express the feeling of the garment. If the garment is designed in such a manner that the waistline is concealed, the placement of the hands at the waistline would likely ruin the line.

There are several basic positions to choose from:

1—Fists on hips with broad part of wrist facing the camera for the strongest effect (in this case, the model must be especially careful to keep the wrist straight—if you bend it toward the camera, distortion will result) fist may be placed with the palm downward, little finger toward the camera with wrist bent downward.

2—Fingers forward, thumb behind the waistline with the heel of the hand sometimes, but not always, against the body. For the longer curve of the arm, let the heel of the hand be lower than the fingers—elbows even with, or slightly behind the body.

3—Thumbs forward, fingers behind the waist—be careful to avoid too much tension in the tendons of the forearm.

4—Variations with the hands placed slightly below

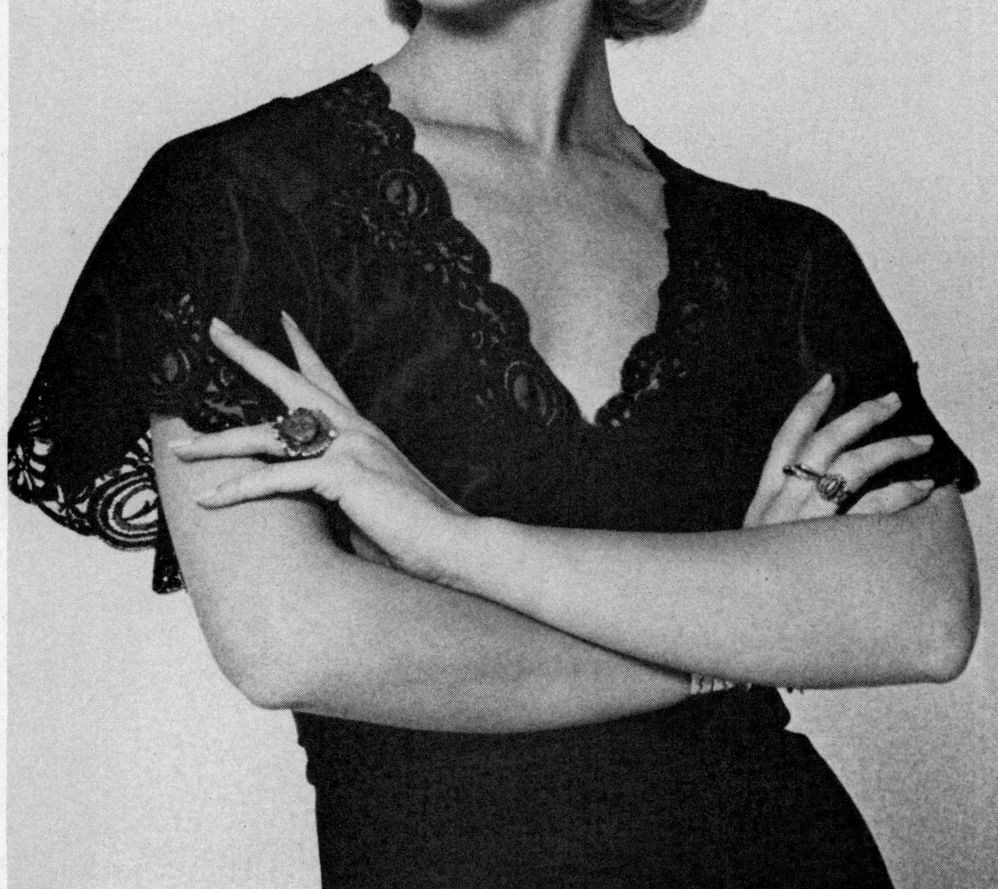

1. Several basic hand positions can emphasize waistline of dress in fashion shots. Fists on hips is one example.
2. Variation with one hand slightly below waistline and other hand placed with thumb forward with arm farther away from camera than body is another hand position that emphasizes waistline.
3. Thumbs forward, fingers behind waist is another waist-emphasizing hand position.
4. Crossing arms can create casual, elegant or sexy effect.

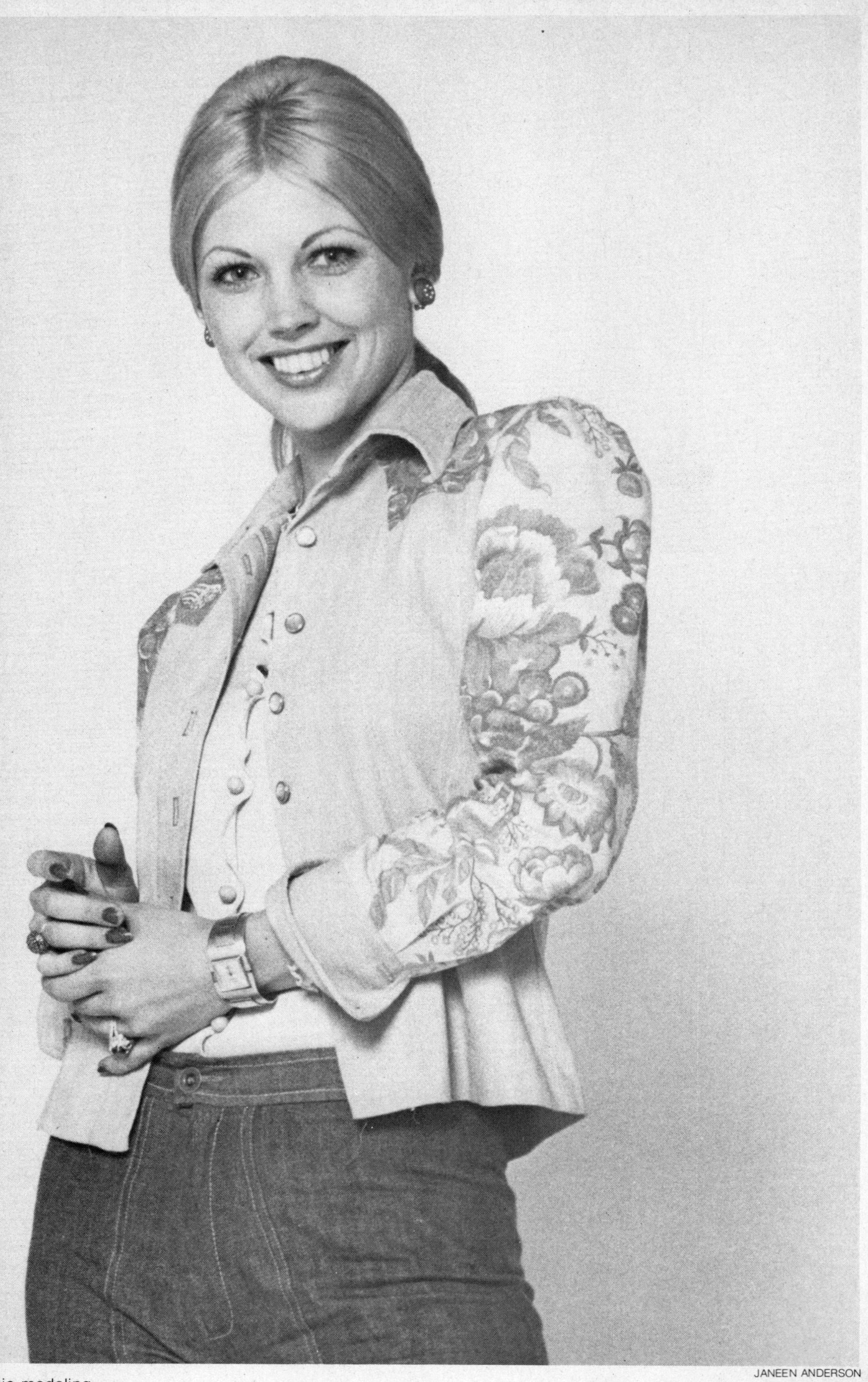

JANEEN ANDERSON

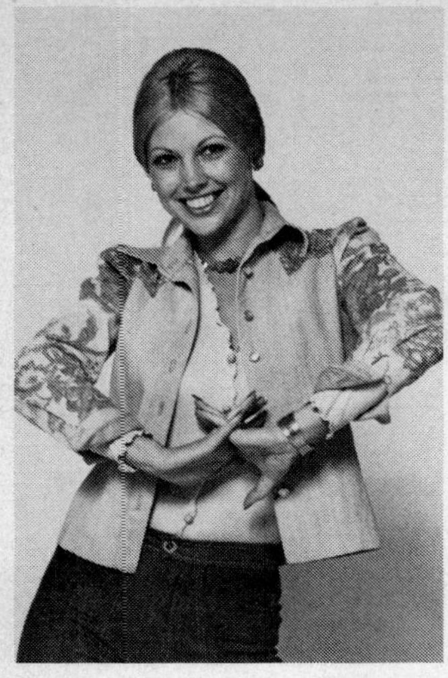

Model touching hands together can produce several effects: casual, cute and gleeful among them.

the waistline or with one hand placed with thumb forward, when the arm is further away from the camera than the body. Frequently the grace and naturalness that results with the elbow back slightly behind the body line more than compensates for the little foreshortening involved.

HANDS TOUCHING—An infinite variety of expressions can be created by a model touching her hands together. The effect may be pensive, cute, dramatic, casual, gleeful—so many different emotions—just with a bend of a wrist or a clench of the fist. There are countless examples of hands touching in magazine pictures. Suggest that your model study them and then experiment with the various feelings and moods that can be conveyed by touching the hands together.

CROSSED ARMS—A model can cross or fold her arms and create a marvelously casual, elegant or sexy effect. Generally, one or both of the hands should be partially or fully exposed to establish definition of the arm direction and to avoid the possible illusion of unexplained bulk across the chest or an armless and handless model.

ARMS BEHIND BODY—For years, it was unthinkable for a model to put her arms behind her body without bending the elbows enough to create definition of the costume shape by showing a little background or light between the elbow and waist. This technique also exposed a little forearm. For special effects, the arm might be pulled in tightly behind the model but be sure there is contrast between the model's sleeve or arm and her body in order to establish definition of the silhouette.

ARMS AT SIDES—Perhaps the most difficult of all hand and arm positions is the simplest in effect—that of just letting the arms and hands drop at the sides. The arms should be bent very slightly with the thumbs at the side seams—never in front of the side seam, perhaps slightly behind.

DANCE MOVEMENTS—The dance can inspire many imaginative gestures. Ballet movements, Balinese or other exotic dance gestures, and especially rock and roll movements all have limitless possibilities. These

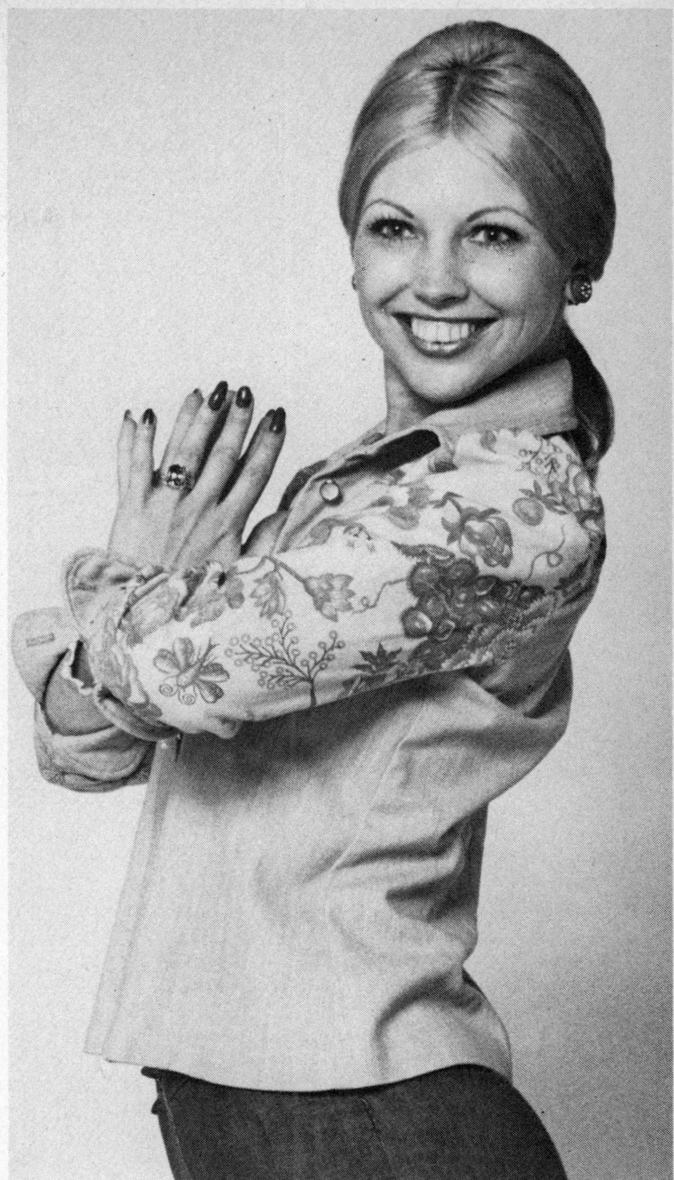

movements are especially popular in editorial sequences. Great action and mood can be created by catching these movements in photographs. Have your model find and try some arm and hand movements inspired by some of these dances: hula, Balinese, ballet, rock, Charleston, modern or jazz.

The preceding section on moods and gestures constitutes a basis of possible movements and arm/hand positions that may relate to the model's response or interpretation of a particular garment, but does not relate to a particular feature or detail of a fashion.

A fashion model quite frequently utilizes a pocket, belt, collar or full skirt to dramatize a detail or effect a feeling of relationship to the dress.

When touching a garment, one should avoid resting the weight of the hands on it or distorting the lines in any way. In some instances, one might vary the natural hang of the garment by spreading out the fullness of a skirt or pulling back a portion of a coat to expose part of the underneath costume but showing the garment to the best advantage is the model's and the photographer's prime concern. The posing, as well as the photographic techniques, should enhance, not sacrifice the attractive features of the garment.

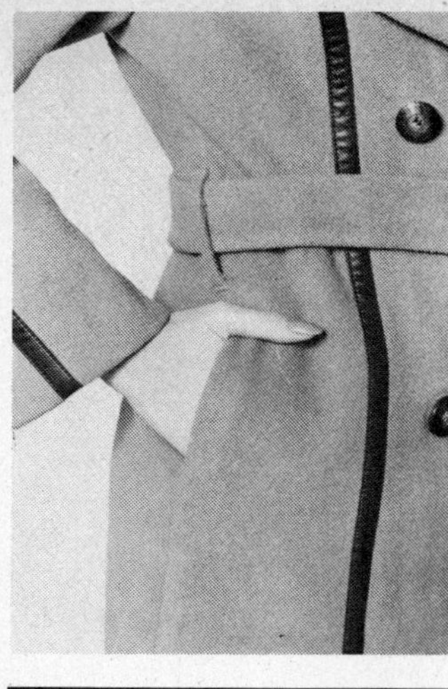

1

1. Traditional technique to emphasize pockets is to put the fingers inside the pocket and leave the thumb outside. Hand must rest against hip bone rather than pull on pocket. 2. 3. Alternative technique to emphasize pockets is to put thumb inside and leave fingers outside. curving wrist.

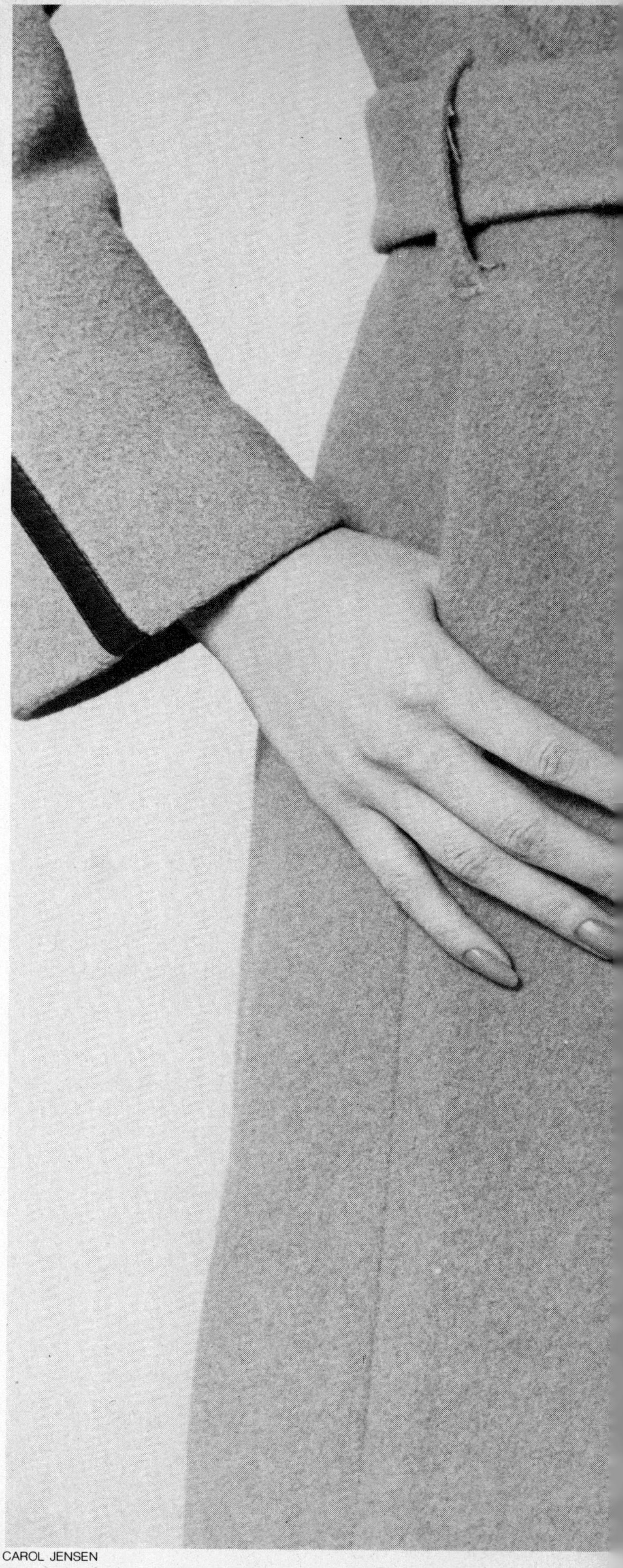

2

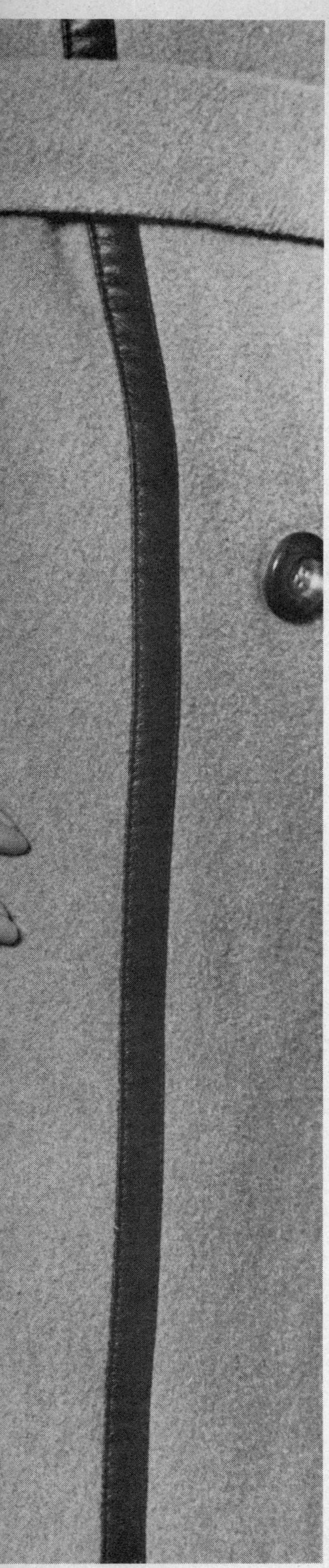

The more stylized techniques of pointing up details of a costume are more often used in fashion-type shots. If a picture is being taken with fashion merchandising as the prime objective, great care should be taken to present an undisturbed garment. On the other hand, an editorial or advertising shot presenting some product or idea other than fashion, should involve less concern for the presentation of the garment.

POINTING UP POCKETS—There are at least three major techniques for attracting attention to, and showing off pockets of a garment. The traditional technique is to place the fingers inside the pocket leaving the thumb outside. The hand must rest against the hip bone rather than pull down on the pocket itself.

The introduction to fashion of narrow, set-in sleeves made the traditional fingers-in, thumbs-out technique sometimes undesirable because it frequently created a strain in the shoulder seam. In this case, as well as when the mood is more casual and relaxed, the model frequently will position her upper arm at an angle that brings the elbow lower (and sometimes backward) with the wrist gracefully curved inward or outward and the thumb lightly hooked inside the pocket with the fingers out. Less frequently, you will find that the model has placed her entire hand (fingers and thumb) inside the pocket. If the sleeve is long, it is quite important for some of the wrist and upper hand to be visible for definition of line.

3

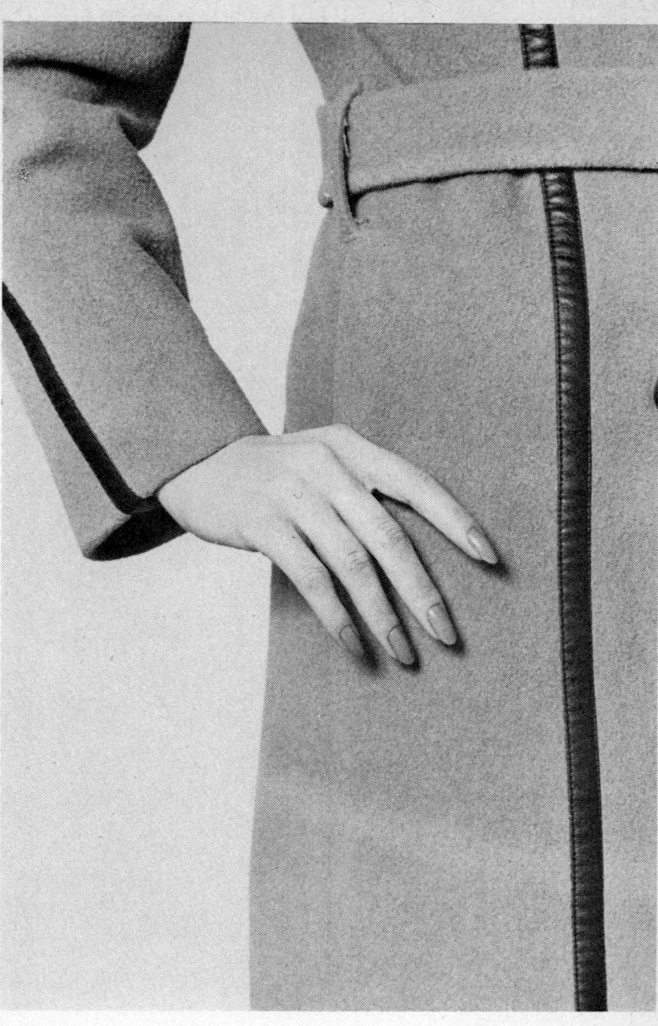

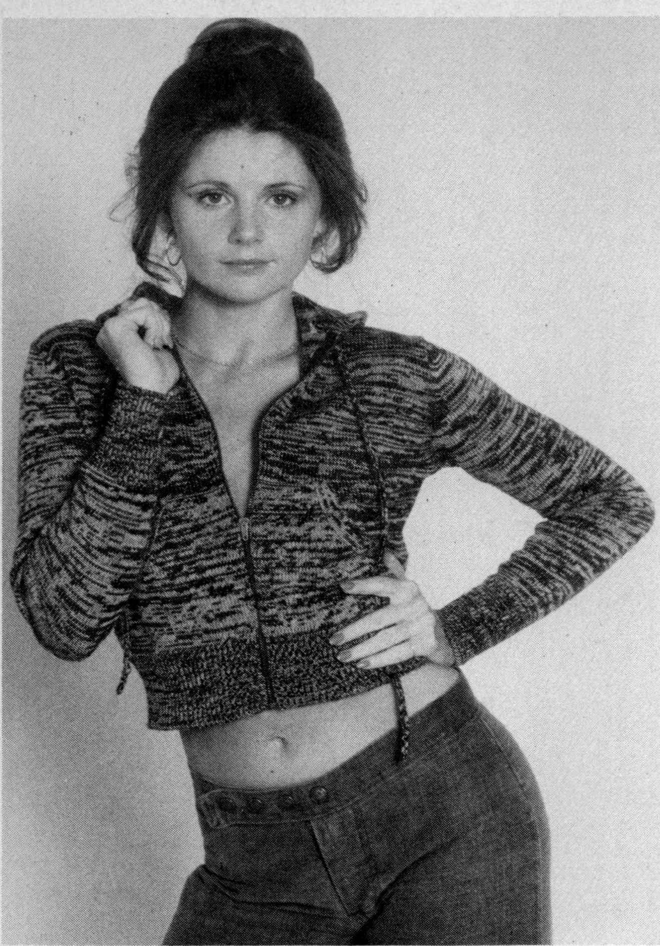

DEBI MAY

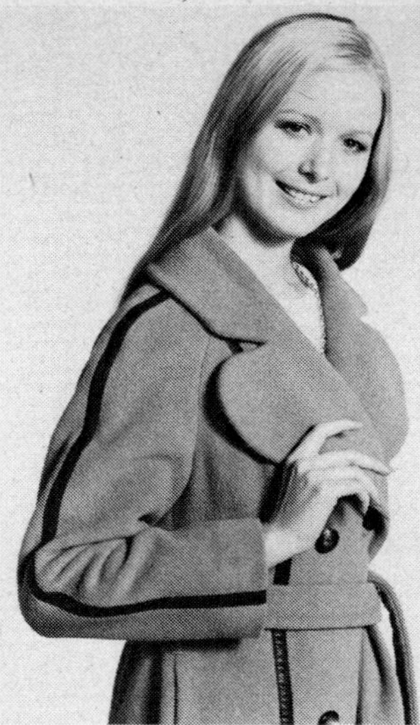

CAROL JENSEN

1. 2. Method of emphasizing a collar depends on type of collar being displayed.
3. An example of emphasizing detail of a garment.

EMPHASIZING FEATURES

JACKETS AND COATS—Attention to a jacket length can be noted by holding or touching the lower edge with one or both hands. If the sleeve line is narrow, it might be necessary to swing the elbow back away from the shoulder line.

An ensemble is frequently shown by pushing one side of the outer garment (coat or jacket) back and placing the hand at the waist or hip of the dress or slacks being shown under the coat. Sometimes models touch the opening of the garment.

Collars may be emphasized in many ways. Touch the front of a high collar (perhaps turtleneck or cowl) with either the fingers spread and pressed against the neck or barely touching with the fingers tapered. Or, show a collar by touching the edge with the thumb under the collar, fingers tapered, with the little finger toward the camera. Elbow can be close into the body or lifted slightly to help define the silhouette of the bodice.

Belts might be made more noticeable by a subtle placement of hands upon the waist or at the hips right below the belt. Chain belts and low hip belts might inspire the model to hoop her thumbs inside them. Sashes lend themselves to all sorts of graceful movements.

FULL SKIRTS—Ladies (regardless of age) respond to the delicious twirls and swirls of full skirts from the time they are toddlers. Action shots quite easily lend themselves to poses inspired by their beauty in movement. Still shots require expertise in handling the skirt. The femininity of a full skirt is generally not enhanced if the model clutches or grabs a chunk of the fabric to hold it out to reveal the fullness. This also has a tendency to destroy pretty folds which are created when the skirt is grasped properly.

The fabric should be held near or at the side seam either with the index and third finger, or with the thumb and third finger. Observe the folds in the garment which are created from the fingers to the hem. They should be arranged to be attractive from the camera's viewpoint.

The model's wrist should be slightly curved with the fingers either following the curve, or bent slightly back to form an S shape with the wrist and finger line.

Unless the model is standing facing the camera straight on with her body, she will probably want to create a backward swing with the arm and hand which corresponds to the hip closest to the camera and bring the other arm forward.

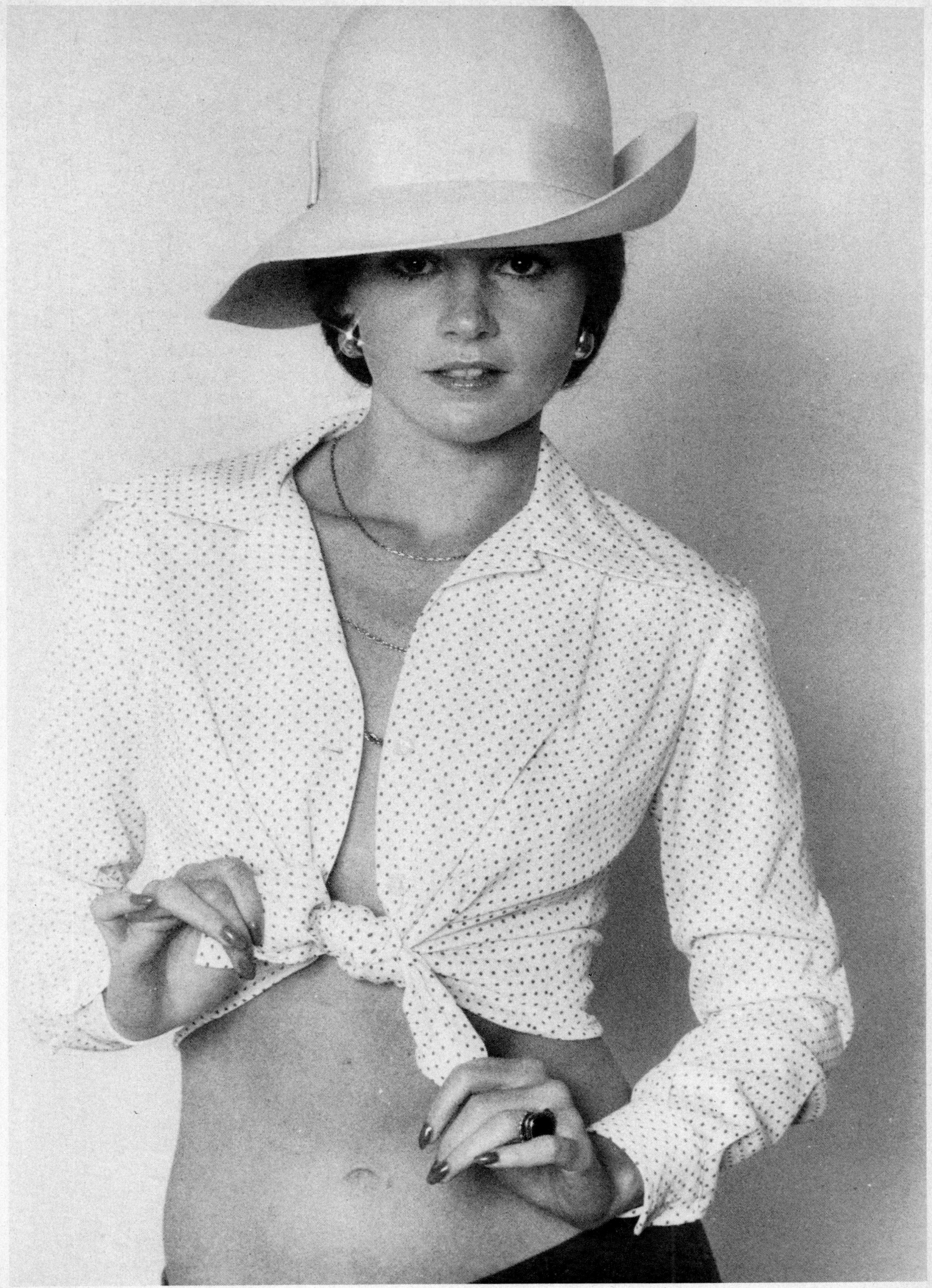

DIANA MAY

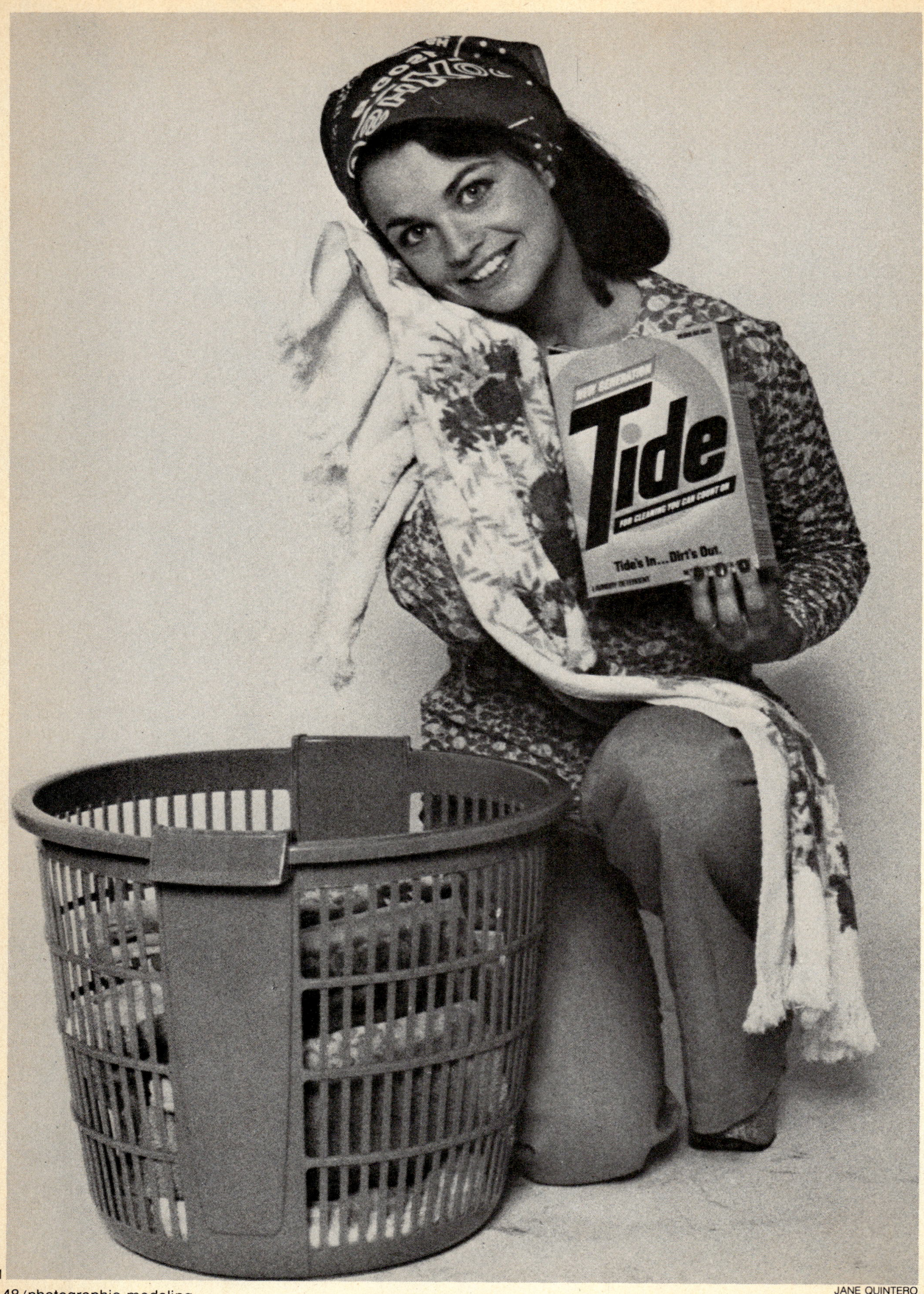

JANE QUINTERO

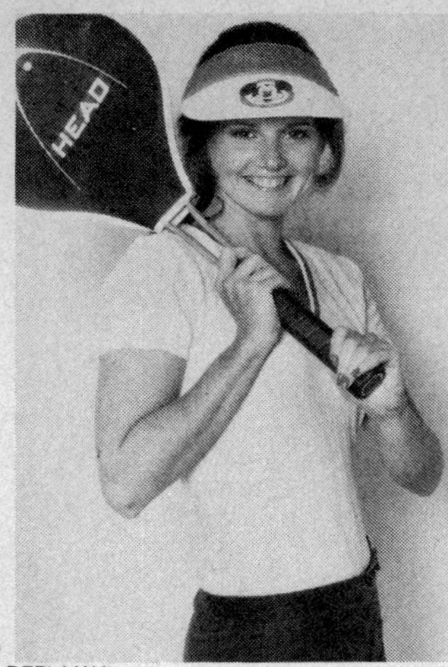

2 DEBI MAY

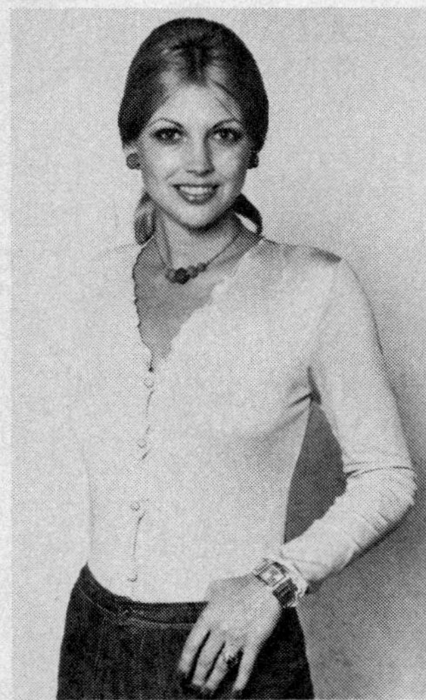

3 JANEEN ANDERSON

1. 2. A product is an item to be sold. and the model is there to draw attention to it.
3. 4. Hands are used to attract attention to beltlines.

This gives movement to the folds of the garment and shows the maximum fullness to the camera.

Quite frequently, the swirls of a full skirt are enhanced by the aid of a breeze, either a natural one or from a studio fan. The model and the photographer may just want to rely on the wind movement, or the model may help it along with swirling the skirt around her. It's important that both the model and the photographer learn to simply let things happen—the unexpected movement of the skirt is almost inevitably more aesthetic and exciting than absolute control of the lines and fabric.

PROPS AND PRODUCTS

Frequently a model is required to hold, use or relate to a prop or product. She must learn how to include these items in a picture with believability and grace. To begin with, it is important that your model learns the difference between a prop and a product.

A product is an item to be sold—the reason behind the picture and the interest is focused upon that specific item. The model is being used to attract attention and center interest on the product.

A product should be held in a position that relates to its use, size and weight, and the hands are placed so that the object is as visible as possible to the camera.

Often, the item is tilted to one side or the other to soften the effect. Shiny objects sometimes need to be tilted slightly to avoid reflections (or be treated with dulling spray). Commercial products frequently have labels that must be fully exposed to the camera. The model should

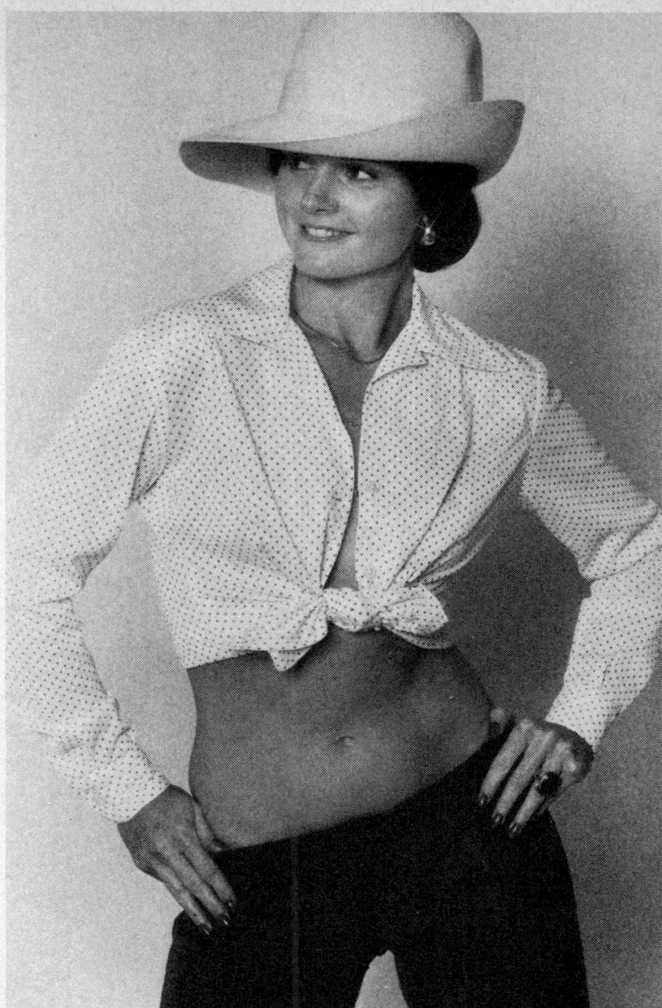

4 DIANA MAY

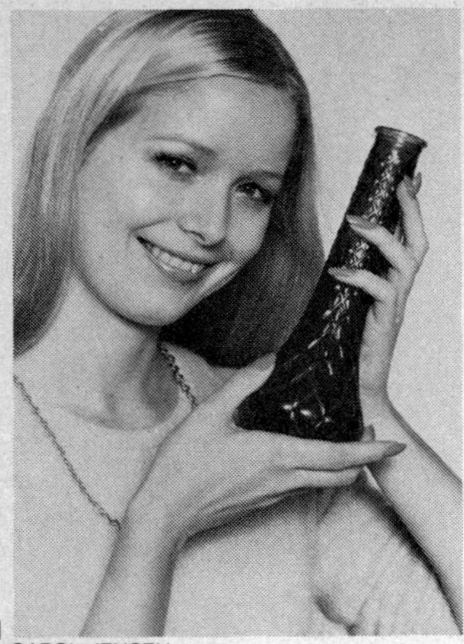

1 CAROL JENSEN

1. 2. A product should be held in a position that relates to its use. size and weight, and the hands are placed so that it is as visible as possible.
3. 4. A prop is an incidental item used to help tell a story or create a mood. Model can either actively use prop or relate to it passively by just holding it.

hold the back of the item with the fingers gracefully arranged so that the label is not covered. Small items are usually held quite close to the face since the viewer's attention is usually attracted to the model's smile—and the item will receive the fringe benefits of that attention. Sometimes it is desirable or necessary also to support the product with the palm of the hand underneath the container.

Models should search through magazines for examples of merchandising shots with models holding products.

A prop, on the other hand, is an incidental item to be held or used to help tell a story or create a mood. Imagination should be applied in the use of props—so many movements besides the traditional use of the item can be utilized. For instance, ordinarily one writes with a pencil—but it

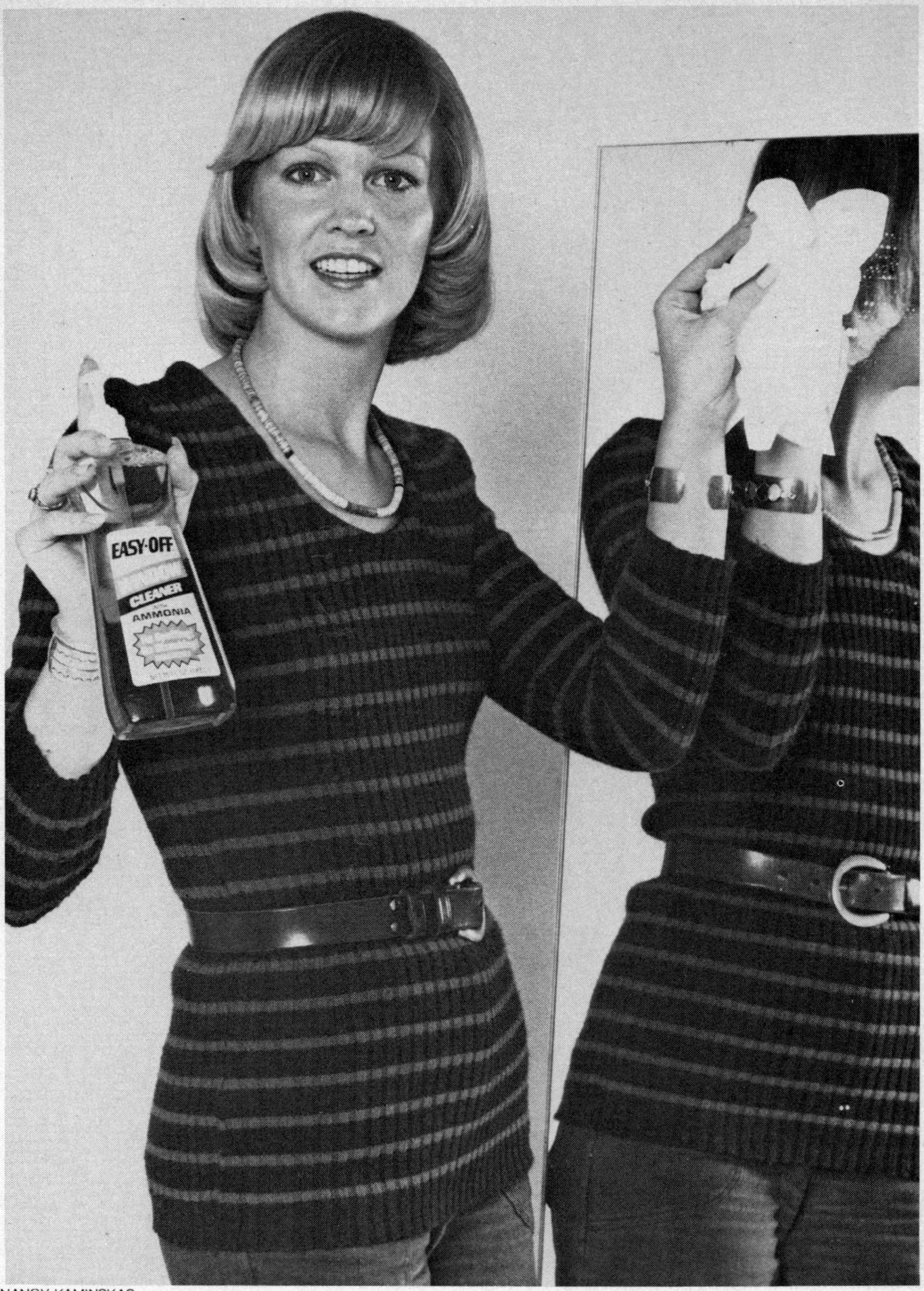

2 NANCY KAMINSKAS

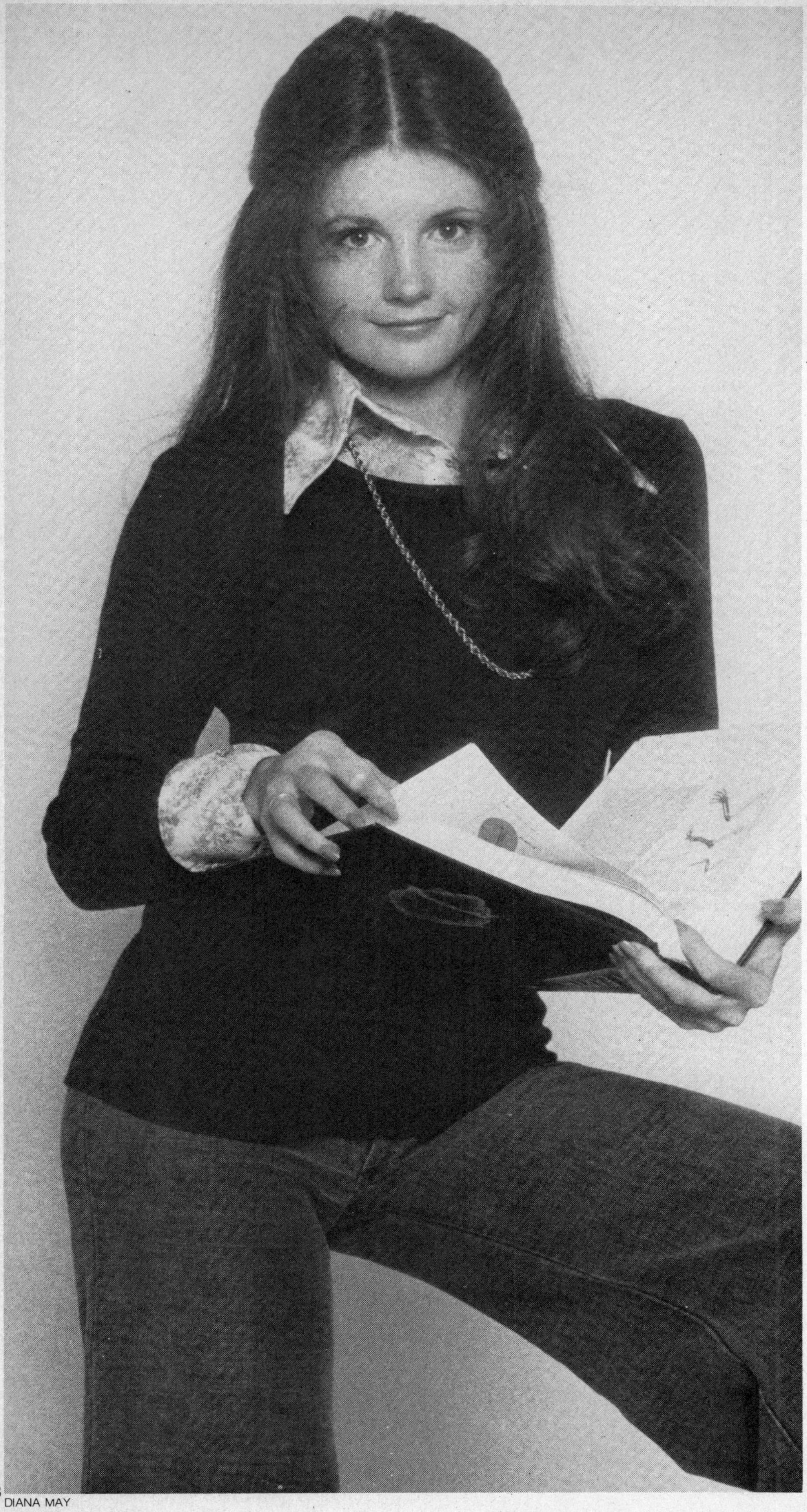

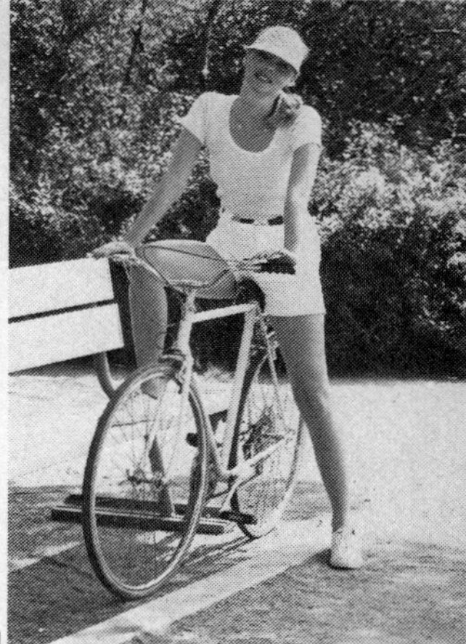
4 CAROL WALLIS

can also be used to thoughtfully rest against the chin or cheek, to chew on; to scratch one's head, or to twirl. Books are generally read—but one can also just hold it, flip the pages or balance it on the head. Stuffed animals can be kissed, hugged, held at the side by a leg or arm or tossed into the air.

A model can either actively use a prop or passively relate to it by just holding the item or leaning against it. The use of props helps to make a picture live—the scene becomes natural and it is easier for a model to assume an unposed attitude. This situational type of shot is becoming a very powerful trend in fashion merchandising and product advertising. ☐

3 DIANA MAY

grooming

The subject of grooming can be a delicate area of communication between the photographer and model. It most certainly can't be ignored but must be approached, when necessary, with extreme tact and honesty.

Refer your model to these pages, and save yourself an encounter neither of you will enjoy. If, in spite of this advice, the young lady still suffers a grooming problem, don't hesitate to be absolutely honest with her.

TO THE MODEL

A good model must be meticulously groomed in every possible sense of the word.

It is important to realize that the grooming program must be consistent—not a spasmodic surge of effort right before a shooting session. Many times a girl may find herself with an opportunity to do some posing for a photographer with very little advance notice so a good model makes perfect grooming a way of life.

Needless to say, a daily bath is in order, but the model's bath should be a beauty treatment as well as a functional cleansing routine.

Consider a lovely scented bath oil to keep the skin soft and smooth and free from scale. The use of a pumice stone on the heels and elbows is helpful unless you prefer the lotions prepared for this specific purpose; in this case they should be used before the bath.

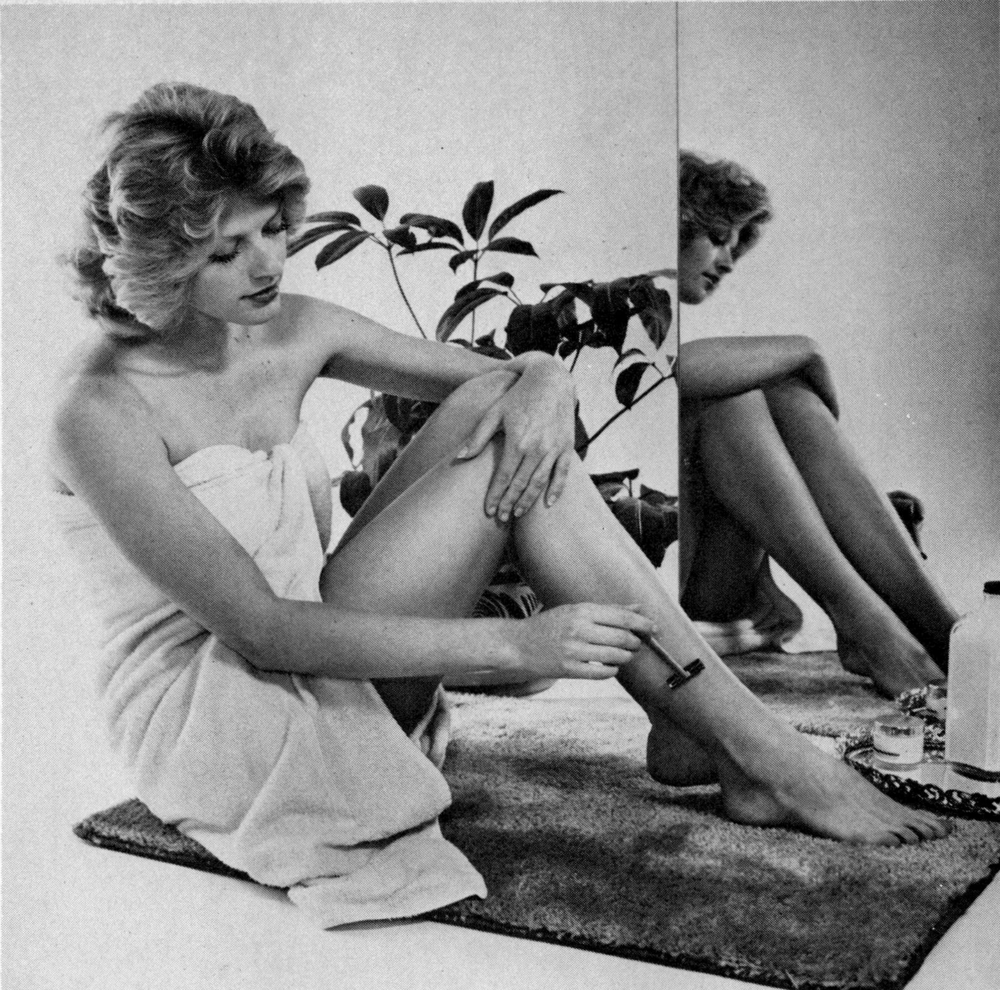

1

SUE FACKLER

(Helena Rubenstein's Pretty Feet is excellent.)

During the bath, you may shave your legs and underarms. The warmth of the bath and the softening effect make it an ideal time for leg and underarm shaving. Many girls use prepared shaving foams formulated for this purpose, or you can create suds with your bath soap and apply it. Consider the grooming needs also of high-cut bathing suits. Any superfluous growth that might be revealed should be removed, either by shaving or by using a depilatory cream. (Helena Rubenstein's Nudit is mild but effective— do a patch test as instructed prior to application of the cream to delicate areas.)

If there is a noticeable dark or heavy growth of hair on the forearm, it, too, should be removed by applying wax or a depilatory.

The skin should be kept smooth and beautiful by the generous use of an after-bath lotion. There are many good lotions on the market. Nivea, Helena Rubenstein, Revlon or Anita of Denmark are good examples. Massage it into the skin so you will profit by the extra stimulation from the massage as well as the lubricating benefits of the

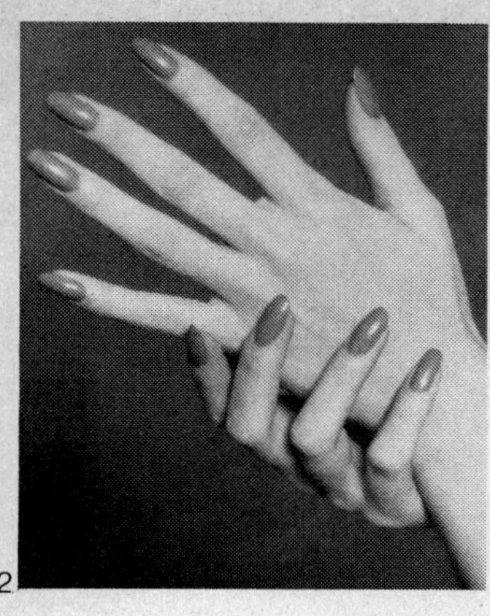

2

*1. Daily bath is in order for models. Legs can be shaved during or after bath.
2. Manicure should include nail and cuticle care, result in hands that photograph well.*

lotion. Apply lotion to the entire body every night, and you will add years of elasticity and youthful glow to your skin.

THE MANICURE

Generous attention must be given to manicures and pedicures. Reapplication of polish very likely will be required before each day's shooting, but a complete treatment should be necessary every two or three days.

NAILS—Shape nails before soaking in water, with an emery board or file made from diamond dust. Steel files tend to split nails. Shape with strokes in one direction only. If you use a sawing motion to shape your nails, it will result in splitting and weakening of the nail. There are many different shapes and each person must determine the one that best suits the hand, the fashion and the mood. Do be careful not to shape down into the cuticle—the nail should be allowed its own shape to the point where the white of the nail starts.

CUTICLE CARE—After the nails are shaped, the hands should be soaked in sudsy water to soften the cuticle. Apply a cuticle softener and push the cuticle back with a manicure implement made for this purpose to loosen and remove skin that has formed on the nail itself. Cuticle clippers or scissors may be used to remove any loose skin, but don't consistently cut around the cuticle.

LUBRICATION AND RINSE—Apply a good nail strengthener or oil and work into the nails very thoroughly, then rinse completely. Nails can be strengthened by a correction in diet or by drinking a gelatin mix. There are also excellent lotions and creams on the market designed to harden and strengthen that may be massaged on the nail frequently (Proteinail is effective).

POLISH—Even the hands of a very young teen model will look nicer with a little clear polish on the nails. Colored polish (shade depending upon the fashion) should likely be reserved for those models of 18 years or older. Most photographers find that bright red or very dark shades or very light whitish-toned pearlized polish photograph poorly.

HAND PROBLEMS—If nails break easily, a triple-coat polish job will strengthen and protect them. Avoid striking tips of nails against hard objects—learn to use the tips of the fingers instead of the nails. Cover freckles with a water-resistant makeup and bleach liver spots with a mixture of lemon juice and peroxide. If your hands tend to freckle, protect them from sun exposure with makeup gloves.

Use rubber gloves to protect your hands from exposure to hot water and apply hand lotion several times a day.

FALSE NAILS—When nails are not of sufficient length or not uniform in length, it is possible that false nails will be needed. False nails should be applied to your clean, unpolished and dry nails. There are two basic types of false nails: plastic and nylon. Both come preshaped and can be filed to suit your tastes. Either type is available in the self-adhesive or regular form. Regular fingernail polish remover should not be used on plastic nails because they will dissolve. Use a special nonacetone remover made for this purpose. Nylon nails are somewhat more flexible than the plastic nail and regular nail polish may be used. The self-adhesive type is the easiest to use but will not adhere to nails for long periods. They come with their own recharging glue to be used when the original adhesive loses its tackiness.

Directions will most likely instruct the user to coat both the real nail and the inner surface of the false nail with nail glue. Wait the specified time so glue becomes tacky and apply nail by working it on with little rubbing movements. False nails are available in slim-line, regular forms as well as shorter nails for a very natural look. Most sets come with extra nails to substitute for lost ones.

THE PEDICURE

Models must be able to slip out of their shoes at any time without being embarrassed by the condition of their feet. It is inexcusable to ruin a picture by the presence of corns, calluses or poorly groomed toenails. Existing corns or calluses can be removed by a podiatrist or chiropodist or you can apply a series of Freezone treatments. This is a product that can be purchased in most pharmacies and is used for three or four nights followed by a hot water soaking. The corn should lift off with ease after that time. Protect the area that tends to form corns with moleskin or callus pads to prevent their redevelopment.

Toenails should be cut with nail clippers straight across with no tapering at the sides, and should never be cut shorter than the flesh of the toe.

After the bath, dry the feet well and work away dead skin around the toenails with cuticle remover and a plastic or wooden cuticle pusher.

Wind facial tissue between the toes to separate them while applying a base coat, two coats of polish and a seal coat. Even if you are using a transparent polish on your fingers, you should use a light shade of polish on your toes.

Legs and feet should be massaged with a good rich lotion every morning and night. □

the
beautiful
skin

Amakeup man or a photographer cannot be expected to become camouflage experts to hide a model's poor complexion. From time to time, however, a photographer may find a model he values and yet she may need some skin-care advice. Obviously, serious skin disturbances should be referred to a dermatologist— but many minor problems can be corrected if the model has a little more information about how to care for her skin.

Cosmetic companies and their inspired advertising phrases have pretty well established a trend of thinking that a lovely skin is the result of extravagant purchases of magic-seeming soaps, creams and lotions. Such a misconception has led many a woman to ignore the important factors of basic skin cleansing.

There are three major techniques for cleansing the face: soap and water, cleansing cream, and cleansing lotions. The selection of the cleansing product to be used should be a careful one. Unfortunately, some of the most popular products are quite harmful and not only fail to thoroughly remove makeup and normal soil, but also rob the skin of its natural acid mantle— sometimes, referred to as the pH factor. More and more, the public is becoming aware of this mysterious new cosmetic term that defines the balance of acidity or alkalinity of the skin.

The acid balance or pH factor of the skin can be disturbed by products that have a high alkaline content. A photographer can gain a model's confidence in his beauty advice if he shows

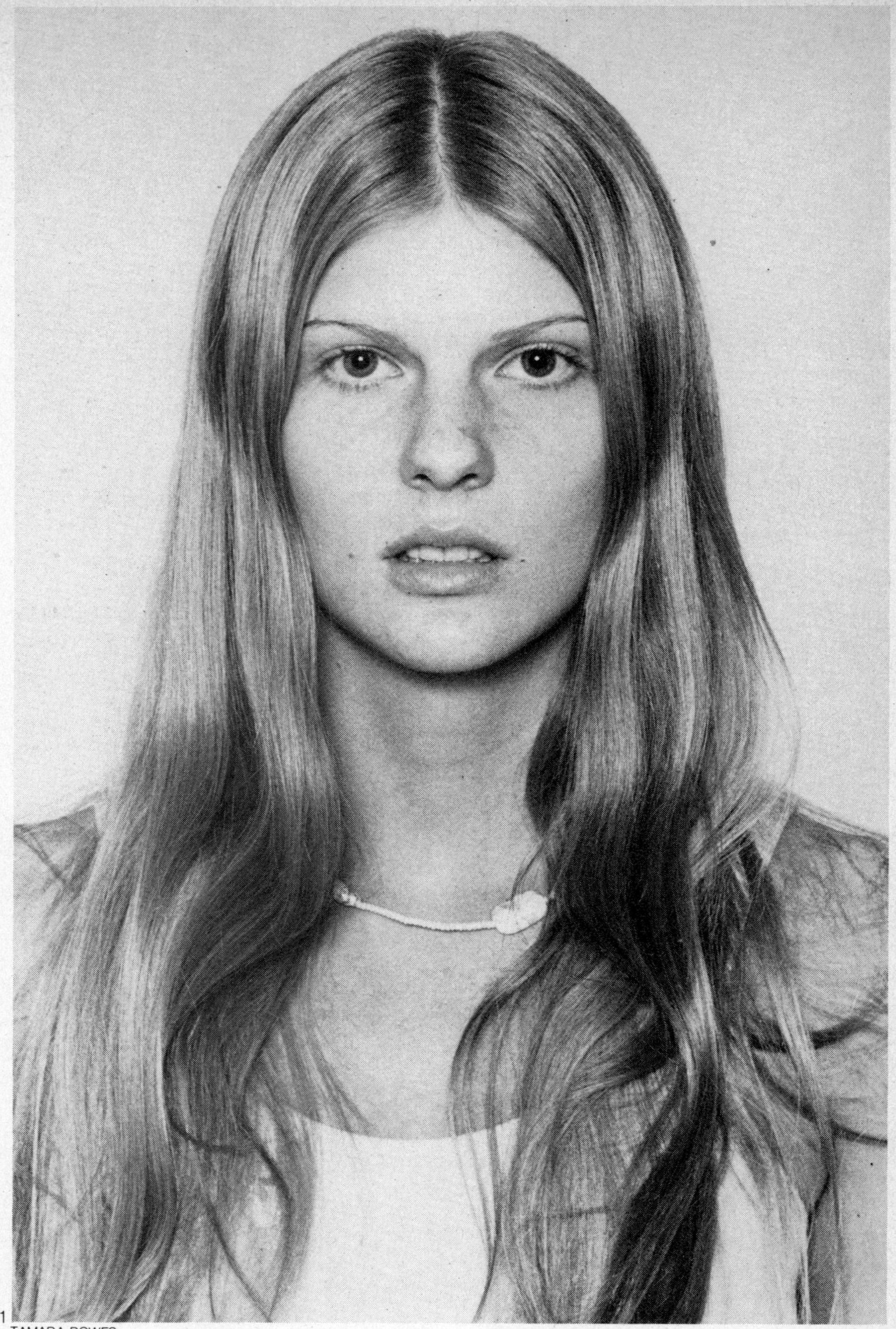

1 TAMARA BOWES

her how to do a simple chemistry test with her favorite products.

Obtain some Nitrazine papers from your druggist—a Squibb Pharmaceutical product. On the outside of the package there is a colored comparative chart. Dip a tip of the Nitrazine paper strip in the cosmetic or cleansing product, shake off the excess and compare the strip to the chart which will give a reading from pH 4.5 to 7.5.

A new baby is born with a perfect pH factor of 4.5 to 5.5, so ideally, any product applied to the skin should be somewhere within this range to retain a healthy, acidic skin that will glow and have a translucent quality. A product that tests into the 6.0 to 7.5 range should be avoided.

Even soap should be tested—moisten the bar and rub a strip of Nitrazine paper against it. You'll discover that all soaps are alarmingly alkaline. There are some beauty bars on the market that are not actually soaps—usually only obtainable at beauty supply stores—and they are considered neutral and won't destroy the acid mantle.

If your model truly prefers soap cleansing and her skin isn't too dry, suggest she try Amino-Pon or Milk 'n Honee—both excellent beauty bars with a proper pH balance. She should use her finger tips to massage the suds onto the skin and rinse very, very thoroughly. (One of the greatest beauty tips you can give her is to advise her to use lots and lots of rinse water.) Extremely hot water should be avoided, but a final splash of cold water is very desirable and will help stimulate and tighten the facial muscles.

Many models find that soap cleansings (or even beauty bar cleansings) tend to dry the skin and prefer creams or lotions. Ironically, one of the least expensive creams on the market is the cleansing product most frequently found in the dressing rooms of motion

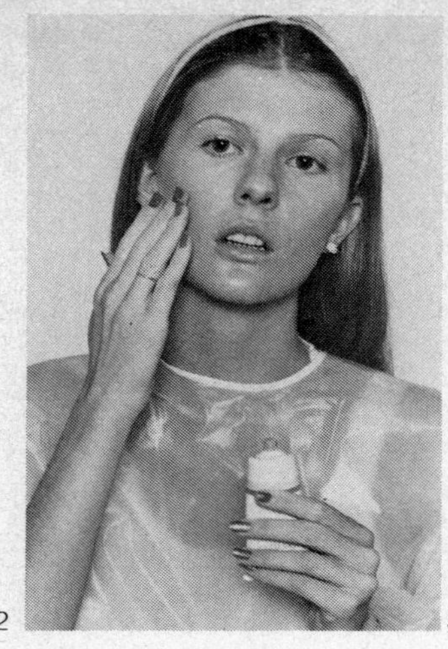 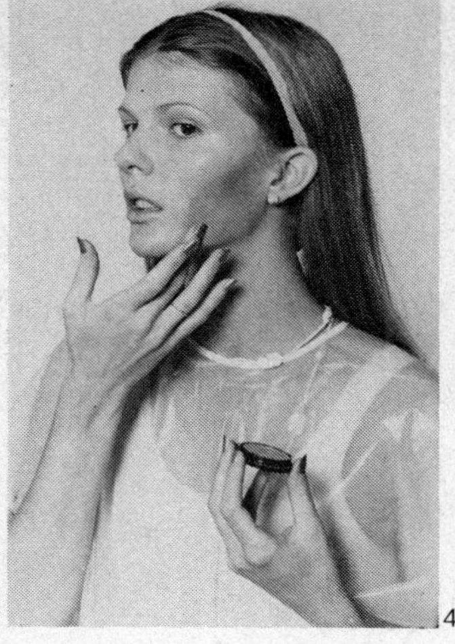 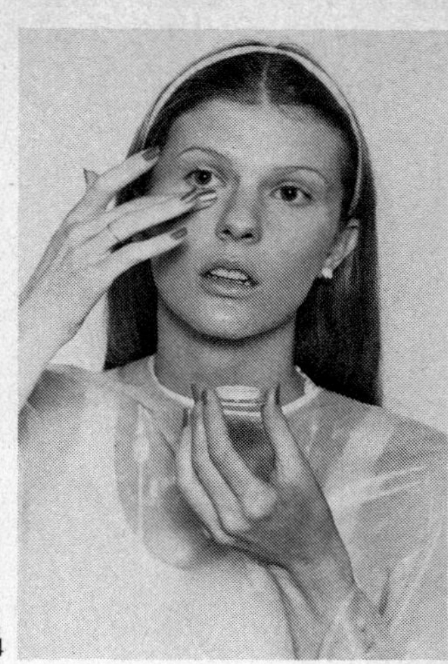

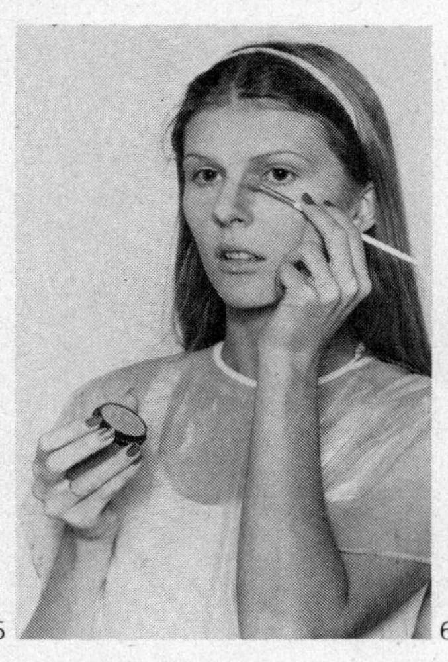 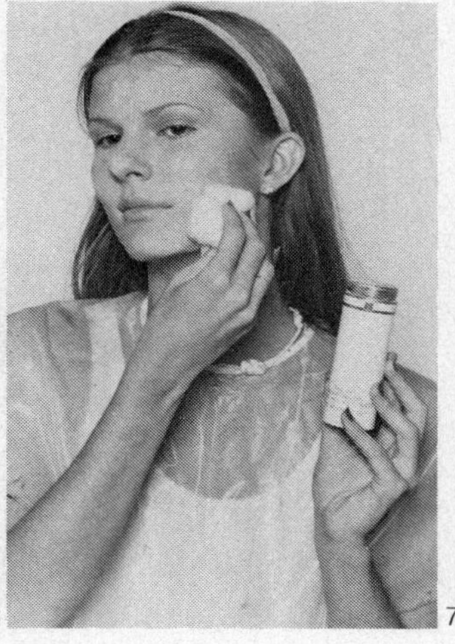 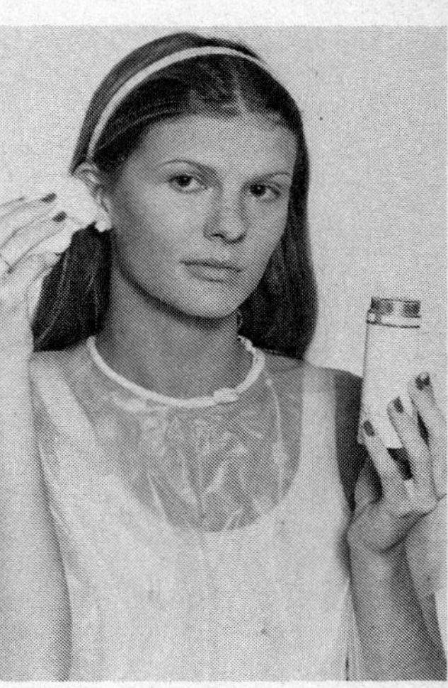

1. Before makeup.
2. Apply foundation base over entire face, and don't forget to include neck and ears.
3. Basic shading is applied as per shading drawing.
4. Lightener applied to cheek bones will catch light for exciting highlights.
5. Corrective shading makes nose appear narrower.
6. Powdering sets base makeup and prevents it from smearing as well as eliminating shiny, too-greasy effect.
7. Use large cotton balls to apply powder. Press powder onto skin with real pressure.

picture and theatrical actresses—Albolene. It's absolutely pure, can be obtained unscented for the girl who may have sensitive, allergy-prone skin and tends to melt upon contact with the warmth of the skin, dissolving makeup and soil. Most cold creams have wax-like fillers which give them a very attractive consistency but detract from their effectiveness. Purchasing a cold cream for its color, creamy texture and/or fragrance is not only nonsense but can be harmful as well.

Nivea is another marvelously pure and inexpensive cream suitable for cleansing and lubrication—very effective (although a bit greasy) for use as a body lotion, too.

Cold cream or cleansing lotions should be applied in upward and outward movements and be removed with a warm, wrung-out

wash cloth instead of facial tissue, which sometimes irritates sensitive skins. Excess should be removed with a skin freshener, or better, witch hazel (inexpensive and pure).

Of course, tissue is more convenient in many cases and the thoughtful photographer will most certainly furnish his models' dressing room with it along with cleansing cream, lip gloss and hair spray, for example.

For the model who wants a good compromise in skin cleansing, with all of the attributes of soap and cream and none of the disadvantages of drying or greasiness, we suggest she try the Creamy Foam

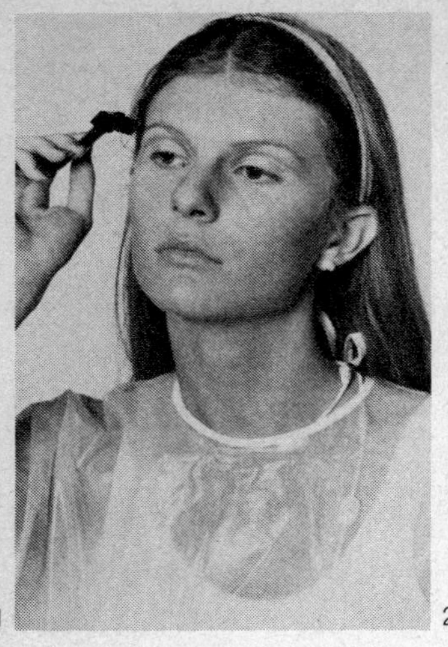 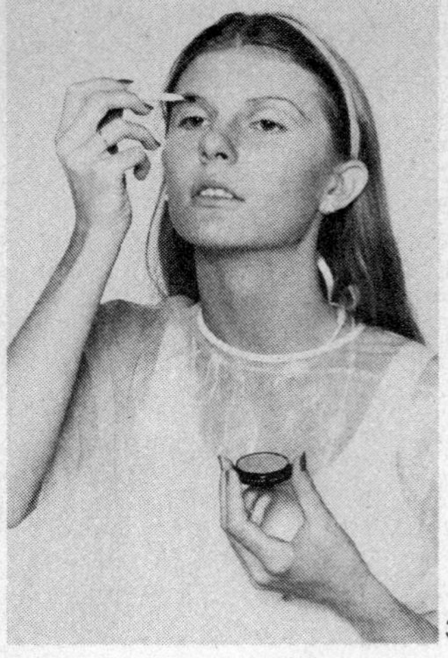 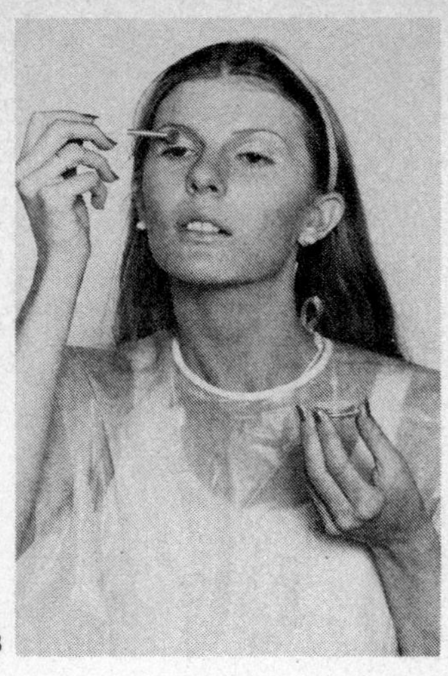

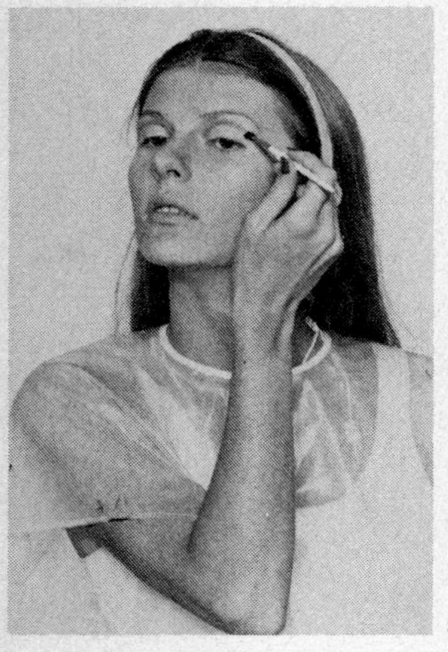 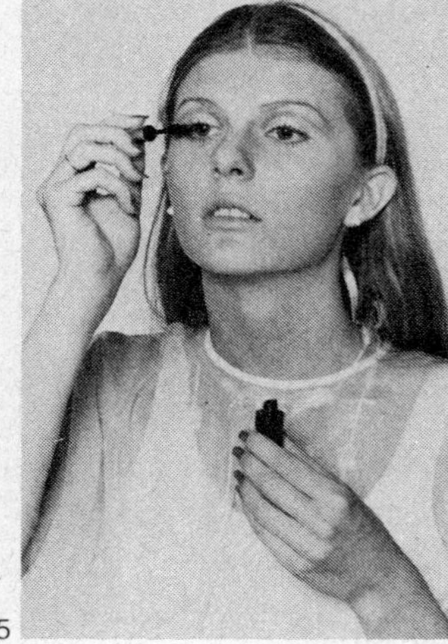 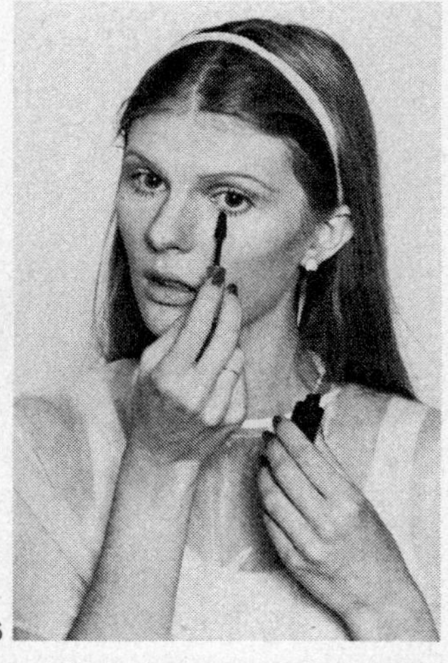

Cleanser produced by Anita of Denmark, available in good department stores and beauty supply houses. It is applied like a cream, then worked into a lather with a small amount of water and rinsed off with tepid water—very effective as a skin cleanser and softener.

If a model's skin is dry, she should use a special lubricating oil or cream, preferably before the bath, so the major job can be accomplished by the gentle steaming of the bath or shower.

Product selection should take into consideration the purest, least perfumed oil or cream possible—test it and smell it. If the model has no need for an overnight cream, she may want to use a

moisturizer—but at any rate, she should at least lubricate the under-eye and eyelid area, around the mouth and on the neck. Any woman over 14 will benefit from this minimal care.

There are special under-eye oils—the use of an all-purpose cream might prove to be irritating to the eyes and frequently is too heavy in texture for this sensitive, easily damaged area. The eye cream should be applied very gently under the eyes, near the laugh lines but not directly on the eyelids. Instead, keep the application of the eye cream to the bone structure around the eye sockets or puffy eyes may result. The model should be advised to avoid stretching the skin in this area since it is extremely delicate and tender.

Cracked, chapped lips certainly don't photograph well and the shrinkage that

results in the lost moisture of dry lips hastens wrinkling about the mouth. Vitamin E oil (not the synthetic Vitamin E—watch the selection) is excellent for any dry area—it is said to help restore skin tissue and is particularly good for around the mouth.

PHOTOGRAPHIC MAKEUP

Male photographers, especially, sometimes tend to think of makeup as a matter totally out of their province. Even some women photographers claim only makeup techniques limited to their own personal needs.

Most experienced, professional models are excellent makeup artists in their own rights. However, whether a photographer is working with a real pro or guiding his own special novice, he must be totally cognizant of makeup techniques and products to communicate the special requirements of each photographic project.

An occasional outdoor assignment with a model who has a flawless complexion—a smattering of freckles, notwithstanding— quite possibly will require no more makeup than a touch of mascara and lip gloss. But most photographic projects require perfection in makeup artistry.

The model's face should first be prepared with a thin protective coating of moisturizer. Too generous an application might result in a greasy, shiny effect so caution your model to be conservative.

The choice of base might take some experimentation and analysis of the model's skin type, coloring, model type and the individual photographic assignment. Most color photography requires a somewhat darker shade with definite pink tones emerging in the total effect (whether it comes from the base, normal skin color or rouge). Black-and-white photography requires a lighter shade—as close as possible to the model's actual skin tone.

Most importantly, the perfect base for photographic work requires

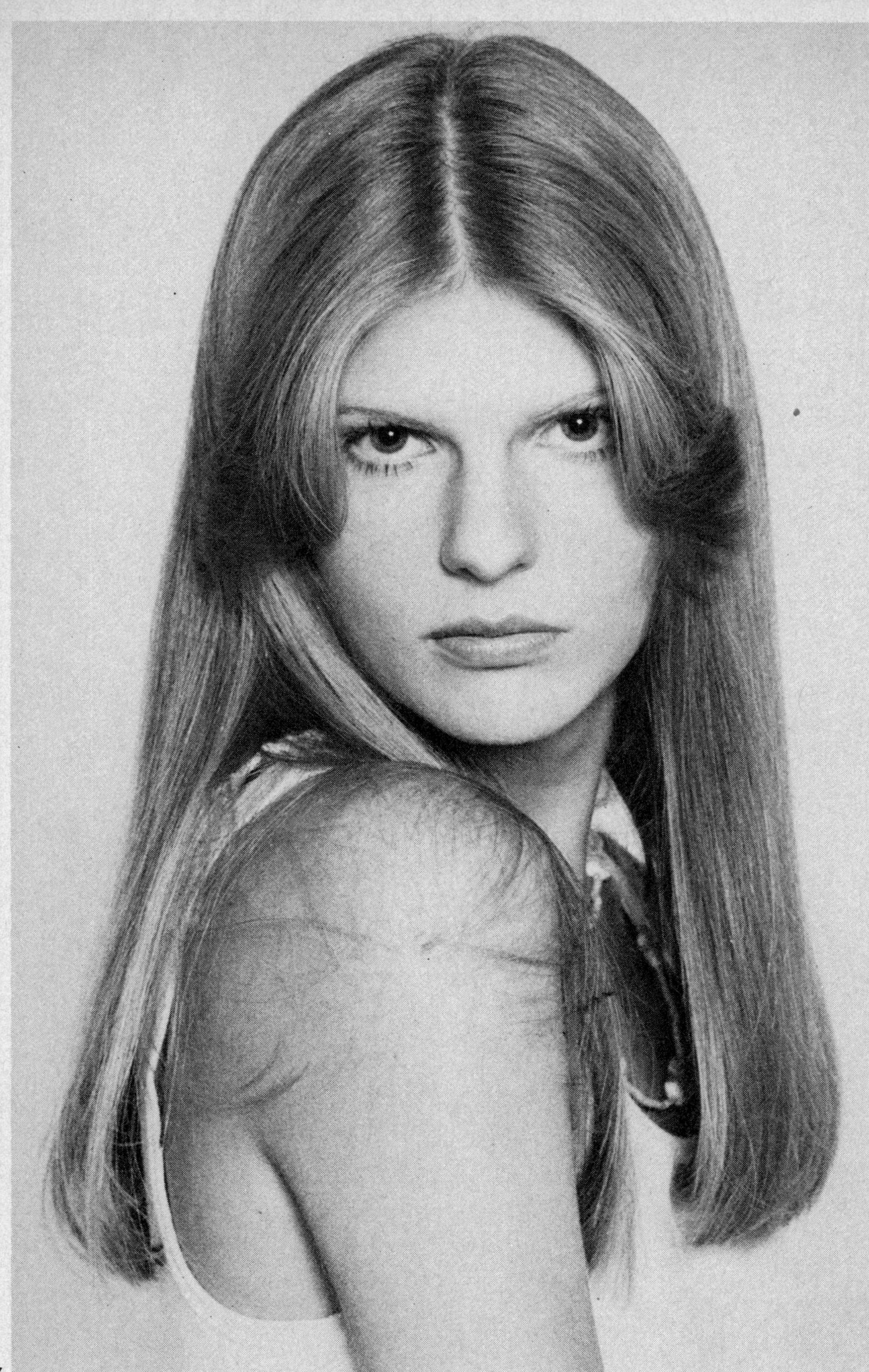

good cover-up properties. Some models use a stick or pancake base—to which there are advantages and disadvantages. The cover-up factor is excellent in these bases, but some girls find them rather disturbing to their complexions, and the end result can be a bit too pasty if not applied sparingly. Most of these products contain colloidal clay (found in soil in many areas throughout the world) and are alkaline in nature. In these cases, of course, the pH testing will be discouraging.

Liquid bases should also be tested. Generally, they are lighter in texture than the stick or pancake forms and usually will not cover up radical differences in skin coloration. Perhaps the most popular of all model's makeup is Anita of Denmark's Make-Up Cream that comes in a tube. It is unique in the sense that it is actually good for the skin, covers up most coloring variations, and comes in a good variety of shades and colors.

APPLICATION OF BASE—Apply foundation base over entire face, and don't forget to include the neck and ears. Work on one area of the skin and thoroughly smooth foundation in that area before going to the next. If you have chosen a liquid, stick or cake foundation, apply by using upward and outward strokes on chin, neck and cheek areas. Always remember not to stretch the area under the eyes or eyelids—it is better to apply foundation to these areas with little tiny patting movements. Foundation is spread on the forehead in strokes that generally follow its line. Use a good sponge moistened in water or witch hazel for the cake or stick forms, fingertips for the liquid.

If you have chosen Anita of Denmark Make-Up Cream,

apply by rapidly patting the face with the fingertips to spread the cream. Don't be alarmed if the cream seems very thick at first—the warmth of the face helps it to spread and one soon learns the correct amount of cream to use. Final smoothing is done in the same manner as with liquid bases in upward and outward movements. Spread soft tissues over the face and apply gentle pressure on the tissue to blot off excess.

SHADING AND LIGHTENING—Occasionally, even makeup foundations with excellent cover-up properties will need the help of lighteners in certain problem areas where the pigmentation is just naturally darker. Ordinarily, the problem areas are under the eyes, on the upper lip, the laugh lines from the sides of the nostrils to the corners of the mouth, and directly under the lower lip. Select a shading and contouring makeup one or two shades lighter than the foundation to correct these variations.

CORRECTIVE SHADING AND CONTOURING—By the use of highlighting with tones lighter than the foundation and shading with tones darker, features can be emphasized, flaws can be minimized, and facial bone structure can be dramatized.

Light shades tend to come forward and dark shades recede. Corrective shading and lightening must be well blended into the foundation, and their use must be subtle enough not to be noticeable to the naked eye. (The camera will see anything the eye can detect.) Refer to the accompanying charts for special notes on the various effects that can be achieved.

BASIC SHADING/HIGH-LIGHTING—Suck in cheeks and apply shading with fingertips (if using a cream

or liquid) or a shading brush (with a cake base) from ear into hollows formed by sucked in cheeks. Eyes will seem deeper-set by shading from top of ear to outer corner of the eye and then up to the temple in a triangle with slightly curved sides.

Use a bit darker shading makeup than the foundation, or reddish brown (mocha) cream shading rouge with cream, liquid or stick foundations. Cake shading rouge may be used with pancake or with those previously mentioned if powder is used prior to shading. Very thin faces will not profit by the use of darker shading in this manner—a lighter shade can be used in the same areas to widen the face.

Aside from the lightener used subtly for correcting facial contour or color variations in skin, pearlized or shiny highlights on the cheek bones, forehead and chin can emphasize contours and catch light for an exciting alive effect. A somewhat lighter shade or a rouge (sometimes pearlized) lighter in tone than the foundation can be used.

POWDERING—After makeup base has been applied and all shading, highlighting and contouring has been done, the next step is powdering. This is extremely important since the powder sets the foundation makeup and prevents it from smearing unnecessarily as well as eliminating the sometimes too greasy or shiny effect.

Regardless of what those attractive, brightly colored ads proclaim, don't use ordinary, drug-store-variety colored face powder— instead stock up on plenty of

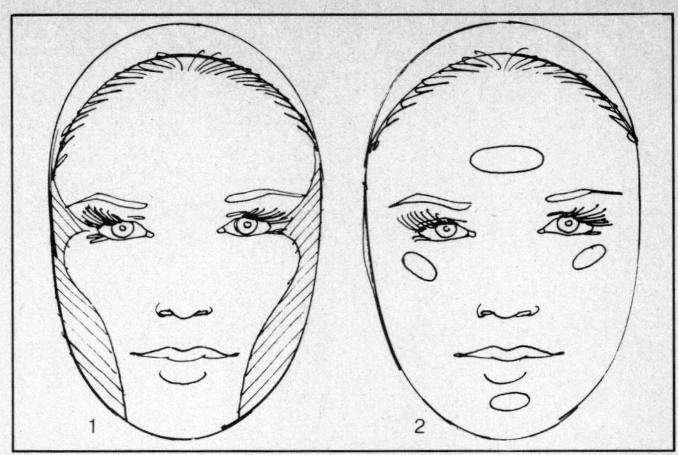

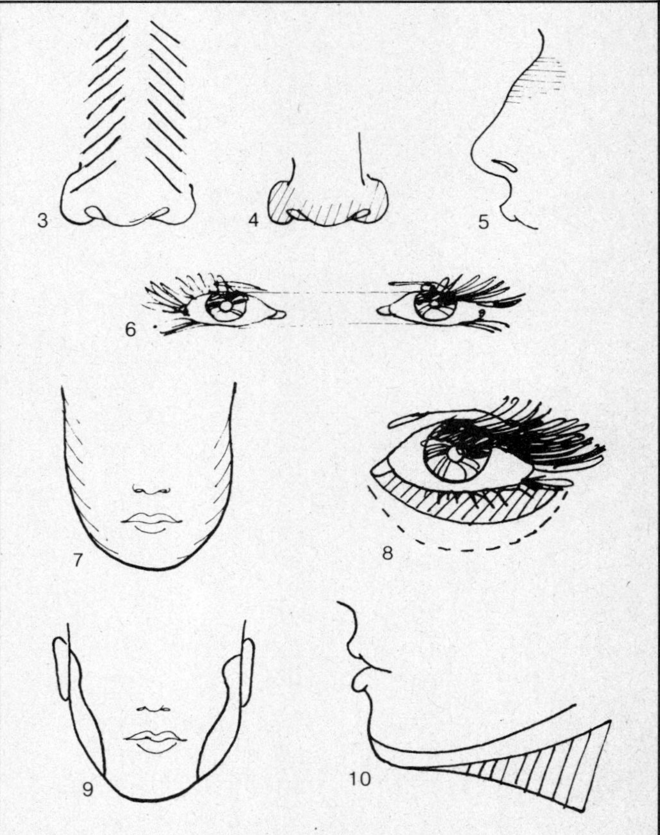

French talc or very fine, lightly tinted translucent powder (avoid white since it will give you a chalky appearance). The French talc is much drier than the ordinary type of colored powder, has greater absorbency and won't cake.

With large cotton balls (never use cotton pads and certainly not a powder puff that will contain dirt and facial oils from many previous uses) dip into the box of powder and press the powder onto the skin with

real pressure. Use powder in great quantities and cover all areas of face, neck and ears, then with other clean cotton balls, flick off all excess. For the finishing touch if desired, you might then moisten a cotton ball slightly with water and lightly touch highlight areas for a light sheen.

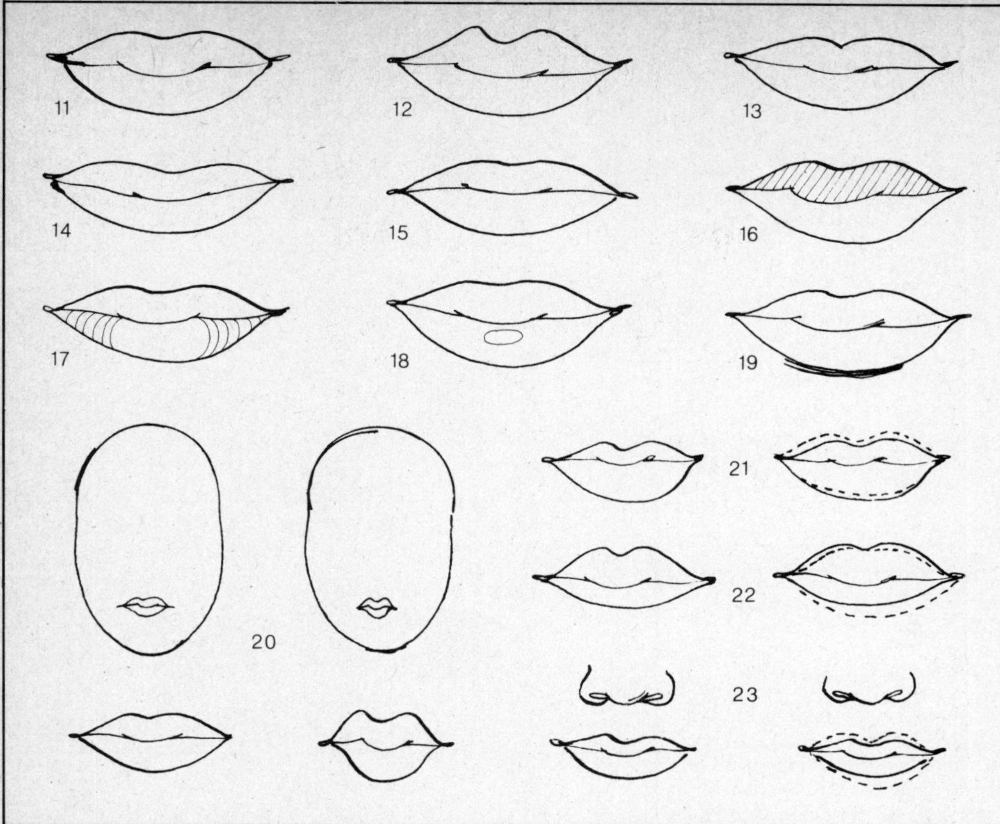

MOUTHS—Mouth shapes and lipstick shades vary considerably with the fashions of the times so a careful analysis of the trends is necessary. The lip chart included here is a basic guide, and a thorough knowledge of the possible shapes and techniques will help make the necessary variations that fashion may dictate.

The use of a good sable lipstick brush is an absolute must. The brush should be held with the thumb and forefinger and the little finger should be braced against the chin to steady the hand. Start the stroke in the middle of the upper lip and draw out to the corners. The lower lip is drawn from corner to corner. Models who find the lipstick brush difficult to master, sometimes prefer the new lipstick pencils. When the outline is perfectly formed, then fill in the color on the remainder of the mouth.

The lipstick shape may be checked for symmetrical line by blotting an impression on a piece of tissue. In general, the width of the upper lip should be the same as the lower lip so to achieve the desired symmetry, compensatory over-lipping or under-shaping might be necessary; but there are many good models who have preferred not to correct an overly thin upper lip line. If the necessary corrections are noticeable, blank out the natural lip line with makeup before applying lip color. It's always a good idea anyway to apply a very sparing amount of powder to the lips before shaping.

LIPSTICK COLORS—The selection of the proper color of lipstick must be coordinated with the assignment, the model's individual tastes and the fashion trends. Frequently,

1. Basic shading—suck in cheeks and apply shading from ear into hollows formed by sucked-in cheeks. Eyes will seem deeper set by shading top of ear to outer corner of eye and then up to temple.

2. Aside from lightener used subtly for correcting facial contour, pearlized or shiny highlights on cheek bones, forehead and chin can emphasize contours and catch light for exciting alive effect.

3. For wide nose, use dark shadowing on each side, highlighting a thin line down the center. Be sure line is thin, not necessarily as thick as the bone is.

4. For long nose, darken tips and sides of nostrils. Don't use highlighting here.

5. For high arch or bump on nose, shade arch or bump, and don't use any highlighting.

6. If eyes are placed close together, use no shading, and apply lightener from inner corner of eye to inner corner of other eye.

7. Mask square jaw by shading from hollow beginning in front of ear and continuing down into and beyond jaw line. Highlight center of chin.

8. For puffiness under eyes, shade puffy part. Lighten the shadow area created by puffiness only. Do not follow basic directions for under-eye lighteners.

9. For too narrow face, darken chin and top of forehead.

10. For double chin, shade entire chin area from chin bone to neck. Draw narrow line along chin bone from jaw bone to chin bone with lightener right above shading.

11. Softly shaped natural lip line is usually best to follow if mouth is reasonably well shaped.

12. Pointed lip line is best on high fashion types, as opposed to outdoor or junior types. It makes a long nose longer and a narrow face narrower.

13. "Clara Bow" or heart-shaped mouth is ideal for '40s or '30s look, not desirable for very full face. Best on a small-boned structure.

14. "Joan Crawford" shape—widely arched, frequently over-lipped—is not desirable for very small faces.

15. Crescent-shaped mouth is best if it happens to be the model's true mouth shape.

16. Three-color lip is special effect. Outline in one shade, use slightly darker shade on top, lighter on bottom. Avoid excessive contrast in shades.

17. Lower lip can be rounded in effect by using darker shade in corners of lower lip.

18. Extra touch of lip gloss or touch of Vaseline in center of lower lip will catch light.

19. Use slightly darker liner on center of lower lip line with a very small mouth.

20. For thin face and short mouth with strong vertical lines, create as much width as possible and soften bows into gentle wide curves.

21. To fix thin upper lip and overly full lower lip, subtly build upper lip and paint inside lower lip line as indicated by dotted lines.

22. If upper lip is heavier than lower lip, paint inside upper lip and over line on under lip, also try dark liner on lower lip and dash of pearlized lightener in center of the lower lip.

23. For especially wide nostrils (which will seem wider with a very wide Joan Crawford-type bow), paint the points of arch closer together.

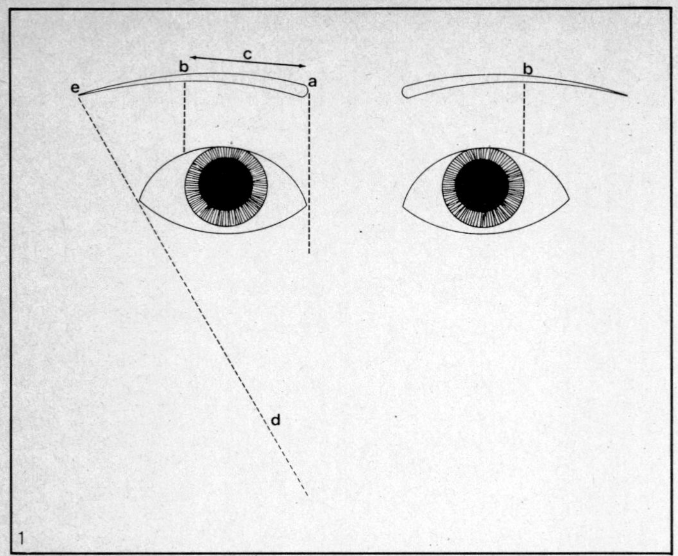

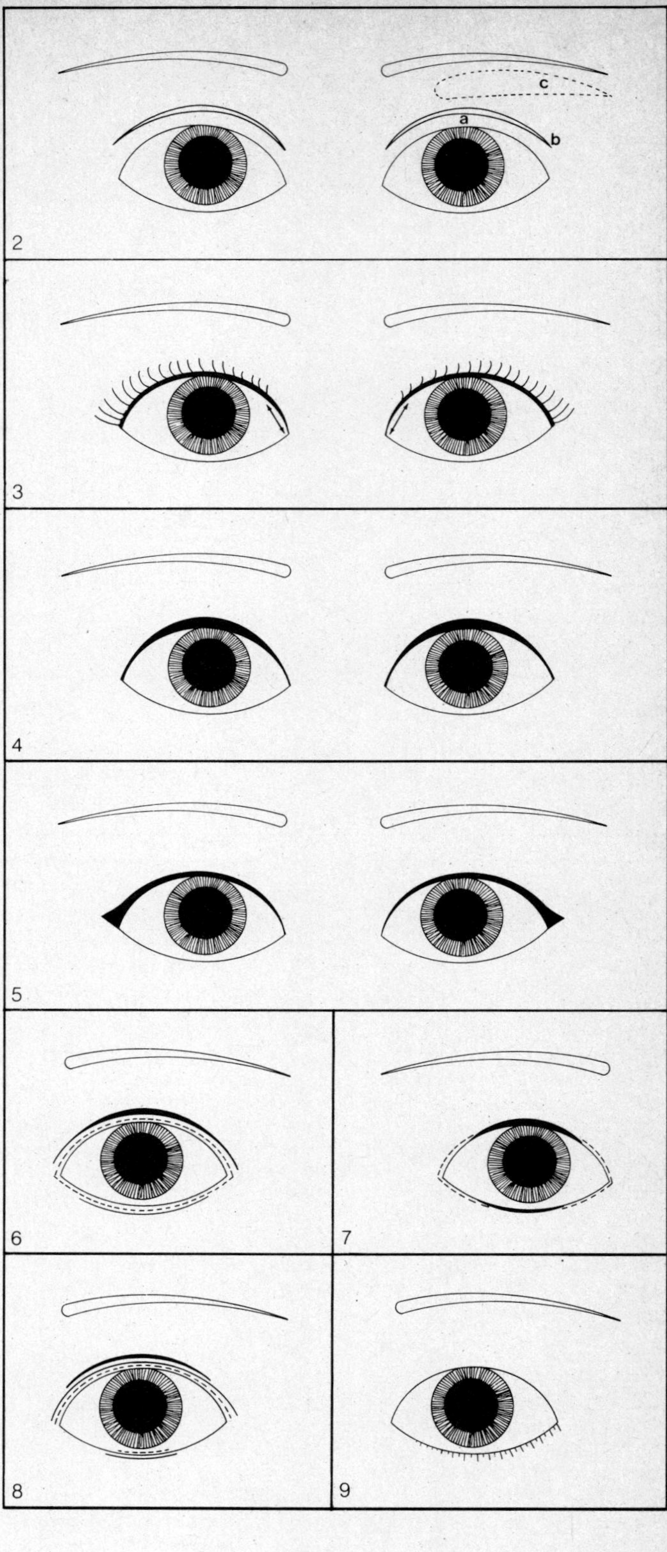

1. For perfect eyebrow shaping: Eyebrow should begin even with corner of eye (a). Highest point of arch should be even with line representing outer third of eye (b). Eyebrow should be same width at its beginning (a) to highest part of arch (b), after which it begins to taper in width (c). (Note: If brow is fuller at beginning than at arch, an angry effect will result. If arch is thicker than beginning, effect will be a worried expression.) Make an imaginary line from side of nose to corner of eye (d). Eyebrow should taper from arch (b) toward hairline right above temple, stopping at point (e). Never shape brow to cut face by having taper lead downward toward chin.

2. Three-dimensional shadow techniques create a deep-set effect. Light shadow—white, silver or very light, sometimes pearlized color—should be in area a. Dark shadow—brown, gray or darker shade of light shadow accent (a)—should be used in area b. Highlighter—shiny or pearlized—should be used directly under brow (c). Brush-on shadow in dry cake form has soft effect, is easy to use. Also very exciting are glistening cake shadows that require wet brush to apply.

If shadow has a tendency to go on in spots rather than evenly, you probably haven't powdered lids adequately.

Use cotton-tipped swabs to correct mistakes or soften color. Never use finger, as oil on skin of finger will only aggravate the problem.

3. Basic eye liner is applied in black, brown or gray. Area from eye corner to beginning of lash growth (arrows) is painted on from below. Then, lift brush above lashes and complete. Eye liners come in three basic forms: cake, liquid and pencil. Most models prefer cake or liquid forms because liner pencils tend to smear. Ultrasoft effects can be achieved by using cake eye shadow as liner.

4. Make eyes seem rounder by painting thicker line above iris of eye as indicated.

5. Eye can be made to seem to slant upward by thickening liner at corners of the eye.

6. Make eyes seem larger and more luminous by applying white or silver liner (both upper and lower, just upper alone or just lower). Black or brown liner may be used above white liner on upper lid, or under lower lashes. Note extensions of white liner at outside corners.

7.8. To widen eyes, frame them with a second liner in crease of the lid (with or without brown crease eye shadow).

9. Drawing lower lashes with liner brush helps widen eyes.

colorless lip gloss is sufficient for a very young teen-age model or in some sporty, outdoor situations. Lip gloss can also be used effectively over a colored lipstick to give an effect of luminosity, and makes constant rewetting of the lips prior to each shot unnecessary. Very light, pearlized lipsticks are not recommended and can sometimes photograph lighter than the skin tone giving a ghastly effect. Bright red lipsticks can be very harsh and will photograph nearly black in a black-and-white photo. Fairly strong pinks, corals and beigy tones leaning toward pink or orange photograph with sufficient density but retain a desirable softness in effect.

EYE MAKEUP—A photographic model's eyes are perhaps the most important facial feature she has. Within the framework of current fashions, she can establish her own individual look through eye makeup.

It's important that the model become aware of the countless makeup tricks that can be utilized. After practicing the various techniques involved, she will be able to determine the look that is best suited to her type and most flattering to her face.

Refer your model to fashion magazines that relate to her type. After studying this chapter she will find it easy to determine which makeup techniques are currently being employed by her particular type for the season.

It's important to keep up on trends. One year you will see heavy liner and eyelashes; the next may go to a lighter touch with very little or no liner and separate lashes to create a more dewy look.

Practice will be the most important factor in perfecting abilities in eye makeup.

EYEBROWS—Remind your model that when shaping and plucking it's important to pluck hairs in the same direction they grow. Most shaping is done by removing hairs below the arch—very rarely above. If makeup

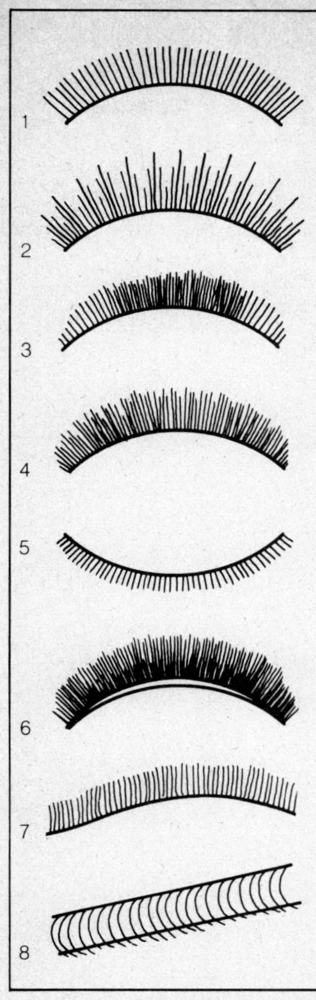

False eyelash types:
1. Unshaped lash.
2. Spiked lash.
3. Double thickness in center.
4. Fringed lash.
5. Under-lash eyelash.
6. Fur lash.
7. Length of eyelash, to be cut in desired lengths and tapered in corners to suit.
8. Roll of separate eyelashes to be glued individually to your own lashes (upper or lower), then cut to length.

styling includes very emphatic lashes and shading, your model could consider lightening the color of the brows with Jolen creme bleach to enlarge the eyes and create a young and vulnerable look.

Urge her to brush eyebrow hairs the wrong way (toward the nose) to remove makeup and loose skin—then to brush hairs into the correct shape. She should try brush-on brow color for the very softest effect. More time-consuming is the lead-type eyebrow pencil. Fine hair-like strokes should be used so that no one stroke is evident. Crayon-type brow pencils are to be avoided.

Junior models frequently find that brushing a touch of Vaseline or hair dressing on the brows creates a fresh, lively effect. Sometimes curly eyebrows need to be controlled with a touch of setting lotion.

One of the most important things to remember is that the basic eyebrow shape is a natural unexaggerated arch. Ordinarily, naturally shaped brows are softer and most flattering; but fashions sometime influence their shape and thickness.

EYELASHES

MASCARA—This comes in cake, cream and liquid form. Some come with fibrous ingredients that build onto the lash to add body and length.

Be sure lashes are powdered and dry before applying mascara. If you're using cake, use just a small amount of water and work it into a thick, creamy consistency, then slide the edge of the brush against the mascara until a little edge of mascara is formed. Then dip the edge of the brush.

In all cases, mascara should be applied in several coats to each lash, taking care that the eyelashes are separated as you brush.

Cream mascaras and those sold in tubes will melt easily under hot lights and are very difficult to control.

FALSE LASHES—These were very much the vogue in the 1960s. The '70s, however, require a more natural effect. Nevertheless, some models and assignments benefit from the subtle use of false lashes and every model should be familiar with the various types available and be proficient in their application.

Eyelash strips should be applied by holding the lash by the hairs in your left hand, with the strip exposed. Use surgical adhesive (preferred) or lash adhesive provided by the manufacturer. Hold the adhesive tube in your right hand. Squeeze a tiny bit out of the tube and touch the lash strip delicately with adhesive. Pay particular attention to the ends of the lash strip. Then curve the lash strip so it will fit more easily on the eyelid. Using tweezers, place the lash on the eyelid as close as possible to your own lashes. Touch up excess glue with eyeliner.

(This procedure does not apply to the eyelashes that are designed to be placed directly under your own. Refer to the directions in the package.)

Lower strips are placed directly below lower lashes.

Individual eyelashes are applied by holding lash or group of two or three lashes in tweezers. Dip them into surgical adhesive or glue provided by the manufacturer. Place on your own lash (near, but not on the root). Cut to the desired length with tiny scissors. Blend your own lashes with the false ones with a very light touch of mascara.   □

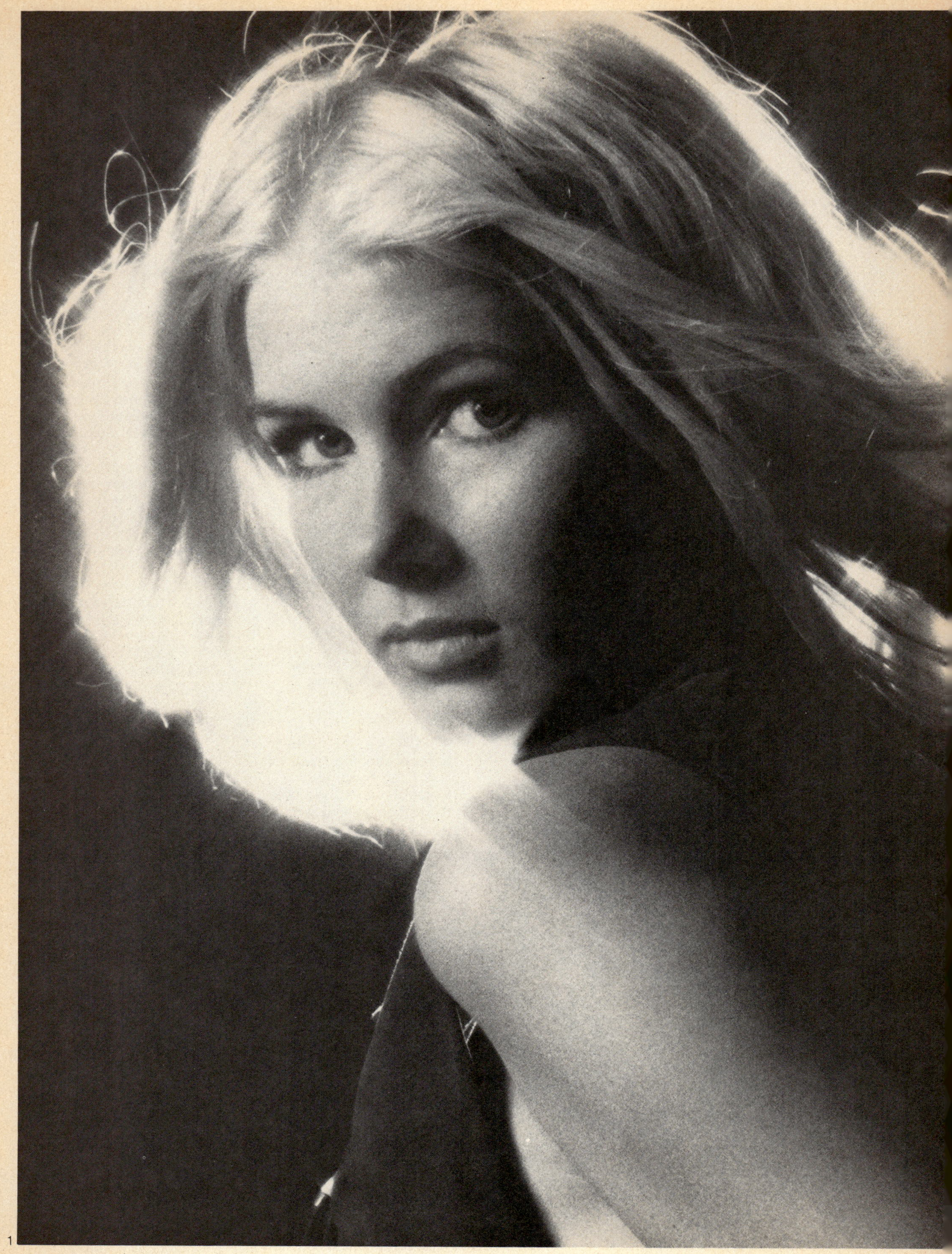

hair care

One of the most important aspects of a model's look is her hair and the styles she creates. Although the model may have an assist from excellent professional hairstylists in her cutting, styling and coloring needs, she still must be an expert in her own right since she is required many times to rearrange a complete hairstyle right on the spot. Before the more artistic aspects of hairstyling can be considered, it's necessary to have some knowledge of the basics of good hair care.

The model's hair needs to be shampooed just as soon as it begins to lose its life and manageability. This might be once a week for the average working girl but a model would be more likely to find that it will be necessary at least every third day. This depends largely upon how many changes she has had to make in the styles on her various assignments (and, incidentally, how much hair spray she has needed to use to hold those hairstyles). Obviously, too, the kind of shooting she has been doing would be an influencing factor. Ordinarily, a day of shooting at the beach or on a windy desert means a certain shampoo that evening.

The selection of shampoo can be taken from a wide variety of good choices.

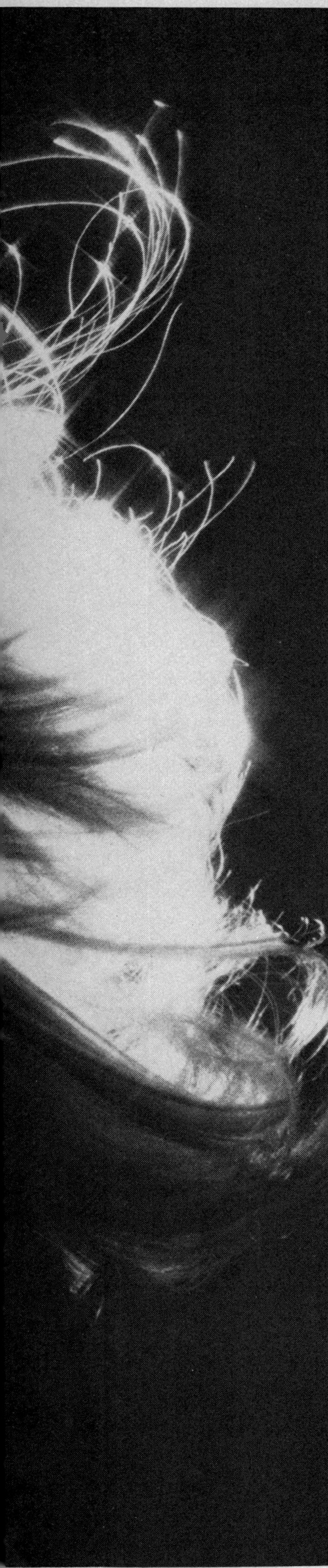

1. *One of the most important aspects of a model's look is her hair.*

Many models favor doing their cosmetic shopping at beauty supply stores that cater to professional cosmeticians as well as the more sophisticated public.

Shampoo concentrates are especially good buys and there are some that are very effective. (Amino-Pon, Milk 'n Honee, Preference, Fermo-Caresse are good choices in either concentrate or regular formulas.) Shampoos should be tested for their pH factors with Nitrazine papers just as one tests other cosmetics. Shampoo should be applied at least twice with a light rinsing between soapings and should be followed with a very *thorough* rinse. Avoid using extremely hot water in the shampoo. Finish with a light dousing of cold water.

The shampoo should include a healthy scalp massage. Press the fingertips on the scalp and move the scalp in circular motions. Work the whole head over thoroughly.

CONDITIONERS

The shampoo should be preceded or followed by the use of a conditioner. Very dry hair might respond well to a Wella Oil treatment prior to shampoo. Steaming towels wrapped around the head will help the conditioner penetrate the hair shaft with much-needed nourishment. P.P.T. by Redken contains polypeptides (proteins) and is a great conditioner that is applied after the shampoo, left on the hair for 20 minutes and rinsed out. Balsam is a somewhat speedier conditioner—just apply and rinse out in a few minutes—or John Redding's Milk 'n Honee Sweet Proteins hair conditioner can be combed through the hair and left on for greater body and manageability.

SETTING PRODUCTS

Occasionally, it is necessary to use a setting gel or lotion to discipline hair that is too straight or too curly or to prepare for an elaborate and definite hairstyle. Or your model might benefit from a very old and popular beer rinse if she has super-fine baby hair. The can or bottle should be opened the night prior to shampooing so that the beer becomes flat and yeasty. It is poured over the head after the last rinse. It is not necessary to rinse out because the brewery fragrance goes away as the hair dries. Remember, any setting lotion or product that coats the hair for more body and manageability tends to sacrifice some of the hair luster.

STYLING

Before the hair is styled, a careful appraisal of facial shape and features is well advised.

There are very few exact face shapes; although the oval face has been traditionally considered the perfect shape, many great beauties have had triangular, heart-shaped, round, square or long faces (or a combination of these shapes).

A model should be aware of her basic facial shape so she can choose hairstyles that flatter her. Remember, it may be difficult for her to be totally objective about a face she has been looking at all these years so the photographer can help her by having her pull her hair back and look into the mirror and analyze her facial shape and features together.

FACIAL SHAPES

OVAL—The oval face is enhanced by almost any hairstyle if there are no facial irregularities to be considered. Generally speaking, all the oval-shape face requires is a soft frame, avoiding any too-high or too-wide effect that might otherwise distort the perfect face shape. Length may be short, medium or long and with or without bangs depending upon fashion and hairline.

SQUARE—The square face needs to be lengthened by height on top and narrowed by softness or curl in front of the ear. Very short hair may prove difficult—long hair helps to lengthen and narrow the facial image. Try these nice tricks: a dip on one side, diagonal part, nonsymmetrical lines. Avoid middle parts and too-flat tops. Fullness at the jaw line or very severe or deliberate lines tend to be unflattering.

ROUND—The round-shape face needs height to slim the face. Too much fullness on the sides or at the jawline might be undesirable. Avoid symmetrical lines that will emphasize the roundness—try a dip on the forehead, a side part or a lift on one side. Don't wear center parts, spit curls or quiches. If the hair is worn short, it should be high and softly curled or poufed around the ears. Long hair can be wonderful but is best if worked with a little lift on the top—lifts at the temples are also excellent.

TRIANGLE—If the face is more like a triangle the hair should be wide and full on top. If hair is worn long, the fullness should be below the jawline—a lift at the temples should be becoming and bangs should be fluffed and wide with fullness on the side of the bangs working into the rest of the hair.

HEART SHAPE—Bangs are nice for heart-shape faces, but don't cut them straight across. Break and/or fluff the bangs—perhaps sweep them over to one side so that a part of the forehead is exposed. Fullness at the

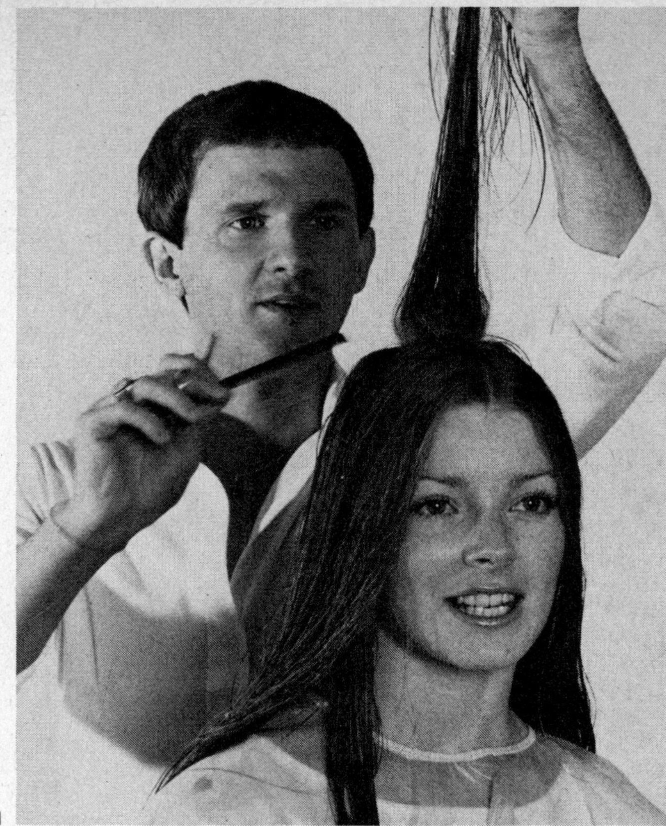

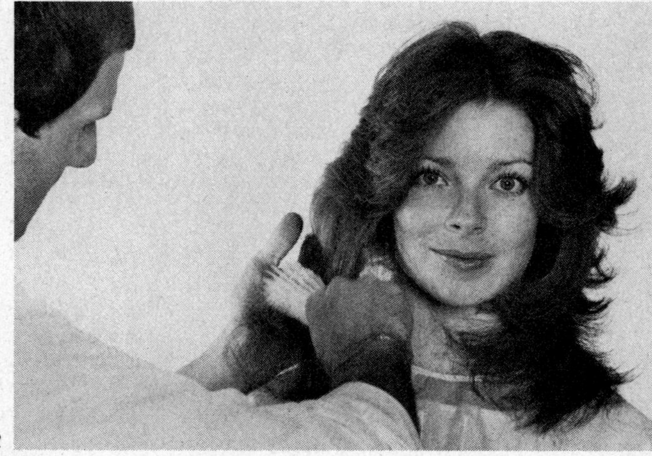

1. 2. Model Deborah Bartlett has an oval face shape. Here, hair stylist Josef McDuffey of David Meyer Hair Concept in West Hollywood shapes her hair into a more current, flattering cut. Cut is tapered so that no setting is necessary—the manner in which the brush and dryer are moved through hair in drying process determines which of many variations of hair stylings possible with this versatile cut will be used.

jawline will soften the pointed chin. Be careful not to wear middle parts and avoid pulling the hair straight back behind the ears, but a little fullness on top is perfectly all right.

LONG—Favor soft styles but not those that are too long or too short. Severe styles are risky—try instead for fullness at the sides. Bangs and low side parts are great. Avoid extra height on top and hairdos that fall in front of the ears. The shape of the face is not the only consideration. One must also acknowledge irregularities in features and learn to minimize them with width and height shapes of the hair styles.

SPECIAL PROBLEMS AND SUGGESTIONS

If a wide nose is the trouble spot, medium to long hair is preferred—but be careful about too-fussy or too-severe hair styles. Don't crowd the face—avoid straight across bangs and middle part or extra width at and directly below the cheek bones.

Low foreheads can be disguised easily by a bang. Start the forward comb of the hair well up on the head.

If your model has a double chin she should avoid fullness about the chin and bring the hair up and away from the face.

A receding chin can be disguised, but be careful of fluffy bangs that add attention to the upper face. Instead, utilize fullness even with the chin line—and be sure to curl hair forward, not away from the face.

When a prominent jaw is the problem, arrange hair with a soft fullness right below or above the jawline and fullness in back to balance—try fluffy bangs.

For the uneven hairline, bangs, curls or soft dips that sweep across the forehead provide a good solution.

Small eyes can be troublesome, so to help them appear larger lift the hair up and back from the temples—avoid curling the hair toward the face.

Attention can be drawn away from a long nose if hair is not pulled straight back from the forehead—it's better if the line is broken with a soft fluff of curls, bangs or a dip on the

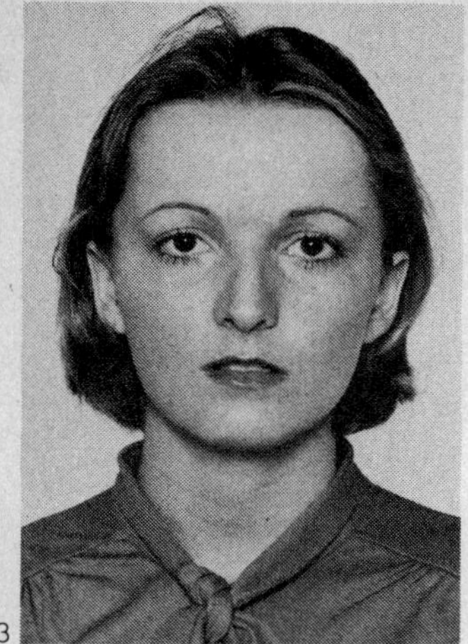

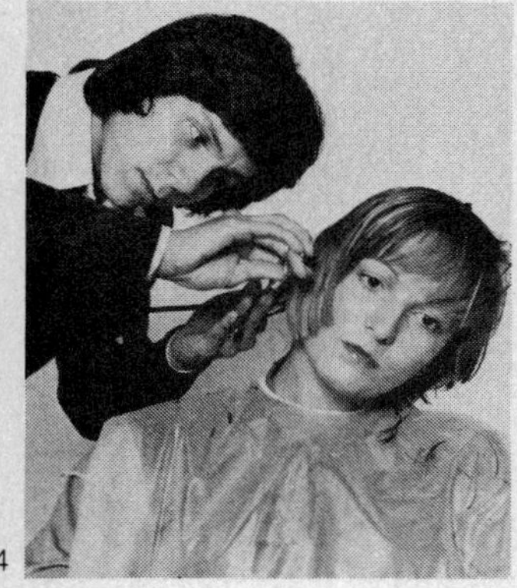

3, 4, 5. Model Diane Tjagvad has classically square face. Square line needs to be softened which would normally be done with height. A too-broad forehead, however, requires attention too. Both problems are solved with a soft, brushed-to-one-side bang, with a suggestion of a lift on top from the brushed-up bang line. Hair style by Sami of Vidal Sassoon of Beverly Hills.

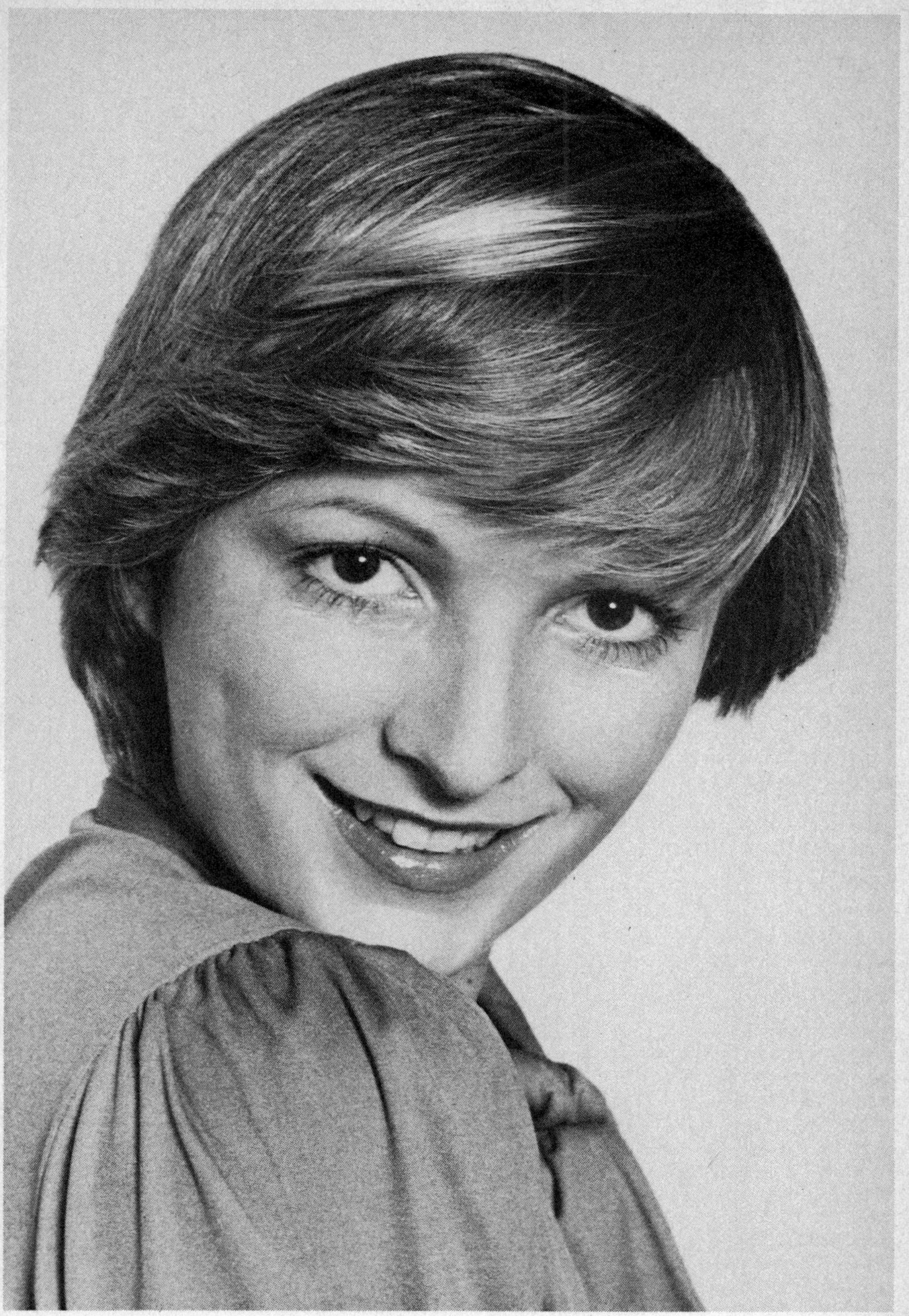

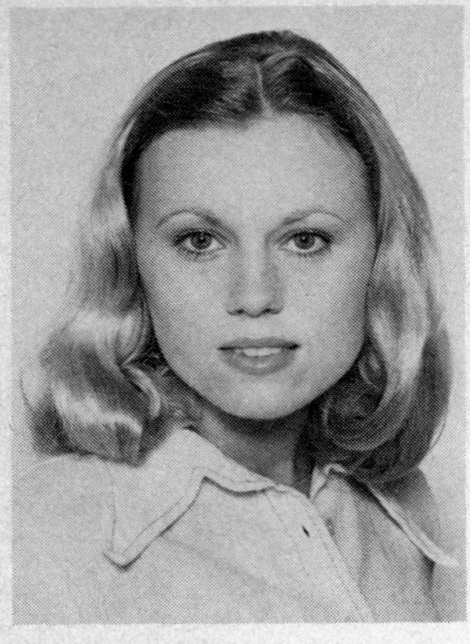

1, 2. Model Joyce Perry has round face, made seemingly ir- regular by too-specific, near- center part and unimaginative, unbroken lines. Stylist Sami from Vidal Sassoon softened her face with a side-swept bang and shaped sides.

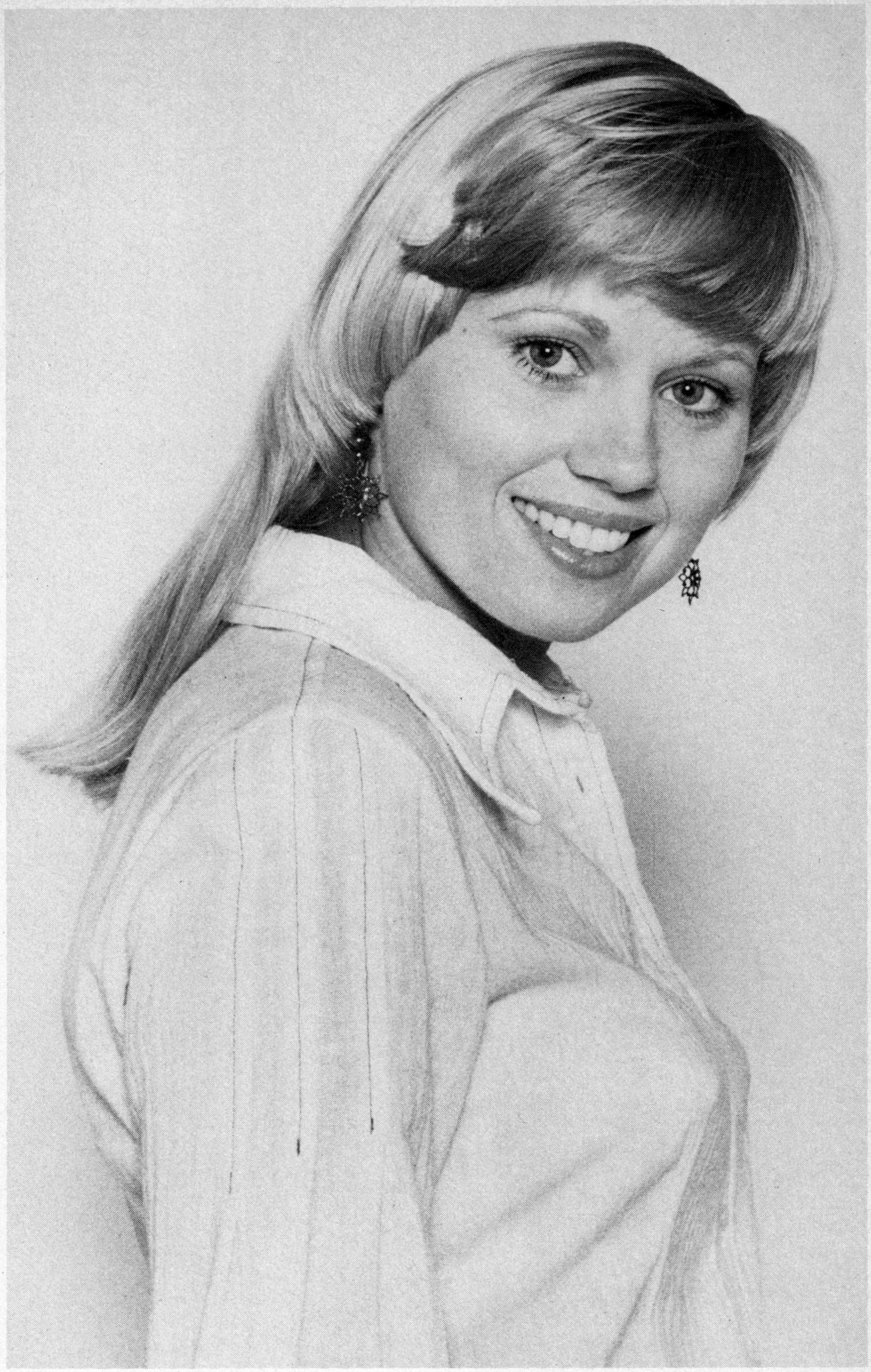

forehead. Avoid severe or extremely short styles.

Hair can be curled in toward cheeks on one or both sides if the model has cheeks that are a bit too full. Cover problem ears with fluff or curl—avoid pulling hair back away from the face.

HAIR COLOR

Before a model pays her all-important trip to the hairstylist, she would do well to have a heart-to-heart discussion with her favorite photographer and consider the color of her hair and whether or not improvement or change is needed.

Some of these color changes can be made easily at home. The more radical changes most certainly will need the help of an expert.

From a photographic standpoint, extremes in hair color (too dark or overbleached) can be undesirable. The hair should never be dyed pitch-black. Some exotic-type girls have naturally near-black hair; but the natural luster and the normal color variations of the naturally black-haired girl make it easier to photograph than hair that is dyed. Dyed

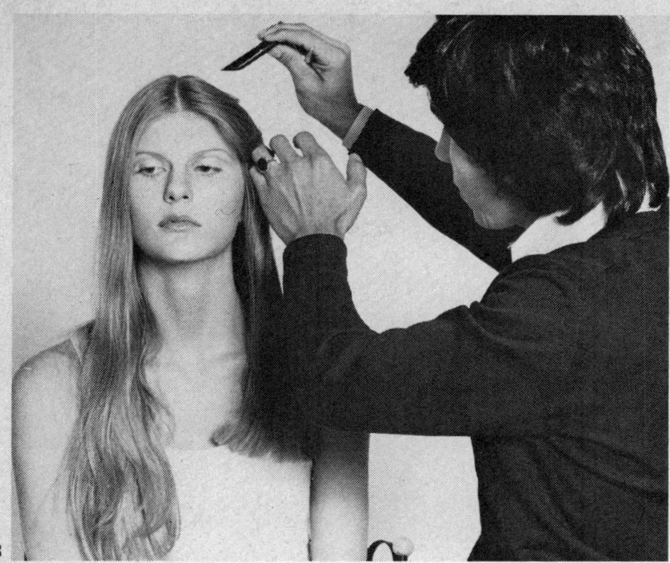

3

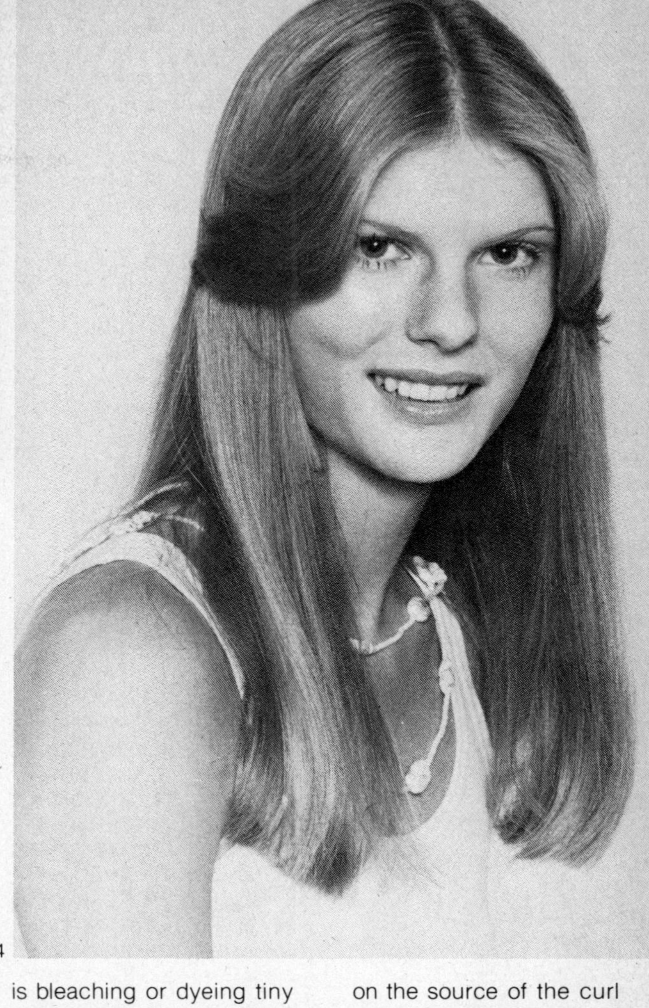

4

*3. 4. Tamara Bowes'
middle-parted
straight hair style is not only
old fashioned but fails to
provide a soft frame for her
heart-shaped face. Sami tapers
sides of her hair to provide
more individuality without
sacrificing length of hair.*

black hair lacks highlights and often photographs like a dark blob with no radiance or definition.

Hair that is too light can turn out absolutely white in photographs and frequently has no tone contrast to the skin. Overbleached hair lacks luster and movement and the necessary healthy-hair-look of a model is sacrificed.

All colored hair requires extra gentle care in shampooing, setting and combing and frequent use of a good conditioner.

HOME-COLOR PREPARATION GUIDE

Rinses are not for radical changes. They can be used effectively to change the shade a tone lighter or darker or to add important highlights. Sometimes rinses can be used to add reddish tones to a natural color or to improve the shade of gray hair. Most rinses merely coat the hair shafts and rinse out in one or more shampoos.

Tints and dyes can be used for drastic changes but must be used in connection with prebleaching or color stripping if the change is to

be drastically lighter than the natural shade. These products do not merely coat, but penetrate the hair shafts. The shade will soften with shampoos and oil treatments but the color cannot be washed out.

You will find peroxide most often used as part of a tint mix (ordinarily 2 parts peroxide to 6 parts tint)—it comes in liquid or much-preferred cream form.

Color shampoos have much the same effect as rinses—they will provide gloss and body to the hair, highlight color, and will generally wash out after a few regular shampoos and oil treatments.

Drabbing is often needed by blonde or redheaded models whose hair color has gotten a bit out of hand and has turned brassy. Use of a white or champagne-colored rinse is preferred. Frosting, tipping, streaking or painting

is bleaching or dyeing tiny strands of hair—it is very tricky to do but is often desirable, photographically.

SETTING TECHNIQUES

Careful and neat hair settings mean smooth and professional-looking styles. The model should towel dry wet hair before setting. The use of a setting gel, lotion or foam guarantees a smoother set sometimes forming a slight crust to give body to the curl.

Major sections and then individual curl sections should be made with the long end of a rattail comb.

FOR CROWN SECTIONS— Hold strand straight up and away from the scalp. Curl should be rolled in such a manner that it can be placed

on the source of the curl strand—not in the part.

AT THE SIDE AND BACK—The strand should be pulled out and slightly upward before rolling.

AT THE FOREHEAD—The strand should be pulled slightly forward.

TYPES OF CURLING EQUIPMENT

Frequently, the photographer requests his model to arrive for the sitting with the curlers still in her

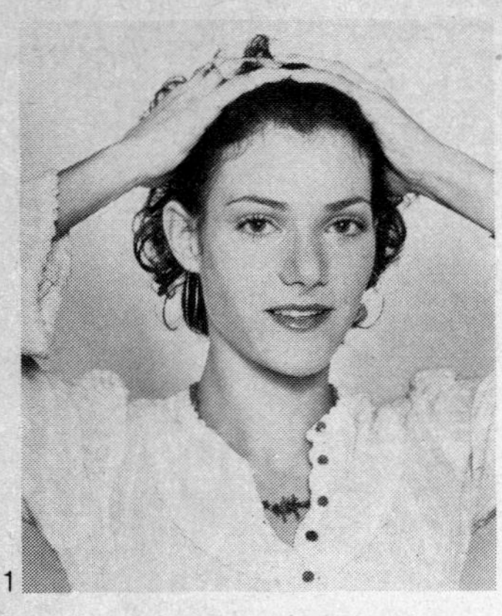

Terry Appell has an exceptionally long face. Very curly hair prevents her from having a style that is flat on top. Sami worked around her already short cut to provide shaping over forehead to break height of curly top and add width to provide fullness. Break at tip of ear tends to cut full length of face in half, and helps shorten line.

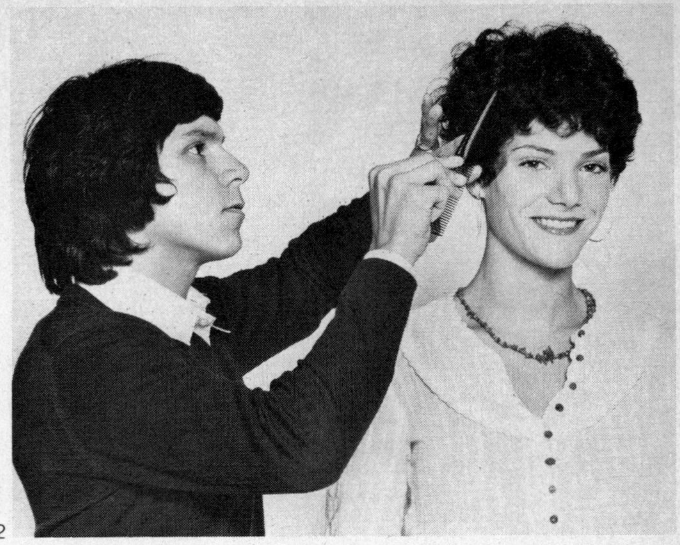

hair—to be combed out at the studio or location.

Even then, from time to time, one or more strands of hair prove to be stubborn and sometimes a complete change of style is desired. The well-equipped professional photographer will have equipment in the dressing room to handle emergencies but if you are a struggling amateur just getting started, you can ask the model to provide these essentials herself.

Curling irons are especially handy for disciplining one or two little sections that seem to be ruining a style, to put in a quick curl or two, or sometimes to temporarily straighten too-curly hair.

Follow instructions carefully and avoid touching the scalp or face with the hot iron.

Electric curlers, steam curlers and chemically treated curlers are preheated by electricity or chemical reaction to boiling water. They have the distinct advantage of achieving quick setting results. Electric curlers are especially popular with models for on-the-spot quick changes or repairs.

Electric blower/curler combinations: Many top stylists no longer set the hair, but set, dry and comb out simultaneously with an electric blower/brush or curling iron combination. They are difficult to master at first, but the results are quick and effects are naturally soft looking.

Magnetic rollers will probably be your model's selection for home setting. They can be used only with wet hair and are not effective for dry setting.

TIPS ON COMB-OUTS

Every photographer should feel confident enough with a hair-brush to be able to make minor corrections in a hairstyle and/or to change the direction of a strand of hair when the model is in place because time, as well as a great shot, might be wasted if she had to go to the dressing room to make her own repairs. The major comb-out, however, will most likely be the models' responsibility.

Even slightly damp hair will ruin a comb-out. Never encourage your model to take her hair down before it is dry unless you can offer her a blow-dryer to speed up the process. Remember, she may very well know her own hair's natural tendencies so if she tells you that the blow-dryer will not work on her hair because it is too straight or too curly, it might be prudent to listen to her.

Rollers, pins and clippies should be removed carefully and the hair brushed out thoroughly enough to break curl separation. It is a common error for girls to brush tentatively in fear of losing the set. If the hair is thoroughly dry, this really shouldn't be a problem and better to risk a little loss of curl than to settle for an amateurish comb-out that shows curl separation.

For a subtle lift at the crown, it's sometimes effective to brush her hair downward while her body is bent over until the head is near the knees.

For a smooth, scalp-contoured crown, brush the hair smoothly over the head, then carefully set some clips in back above the nape of the neck and spray lightly. When the spray is dry, shake the head well and start to shape the style.

To turn the ends up, place the hand on top of the hair and brush ends up and over the hand.

To turn the ends under, place the hand under the hair and brush the ends under the edge of the hand.

Hair separation or awry hair sometimes needs to be disciplined with a little teasing or back-combing. Complete back-combing all over the scalp was, at one time, the preparation for

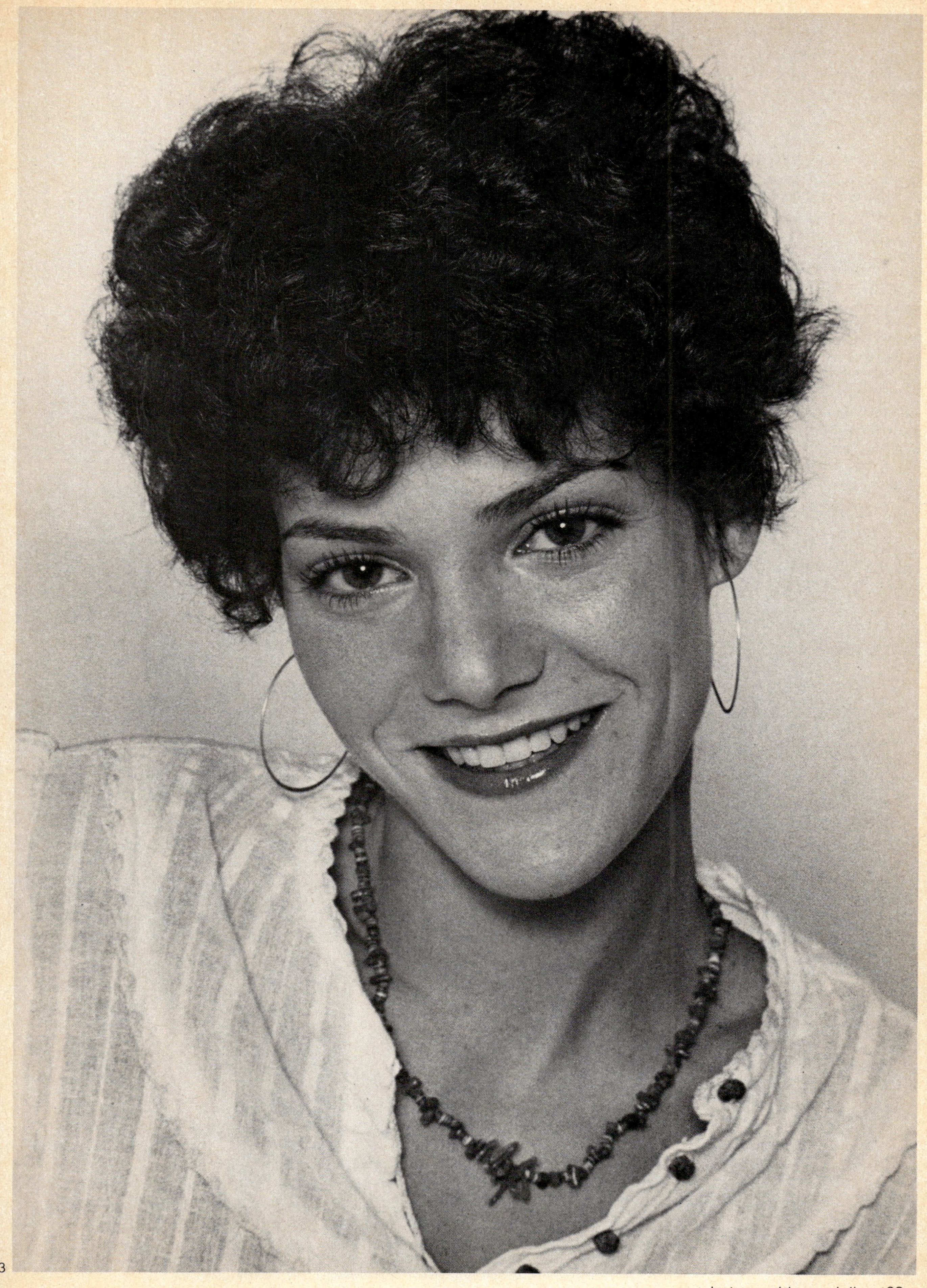

nearly every hair style. It is less frequently used in such an unlimited sense in the fashions of the '70s. But discretionary use of this technique can work wonders with otherwise unmanageable hair or sections of hair and every model *and* photographer should master the technique.

BACK-COMBING OR TEASING—The only equipment necessary is a narrow styling or teasing brush or a teasing comb which has varied-length teeth (usually rattail):

For height at the crown, grasp slim strands no more than an inch wide starting at the very back of the crown. Hold strand firmly and straight up from the crown, brush or comb hair towards the scalp deliberately tangling the hair, with the greatest tangle close to the scalp. When the section requiring the lift has been teased to the degree desired, smooth over the teased section with a brush, starting at the ends and using a very light touch.

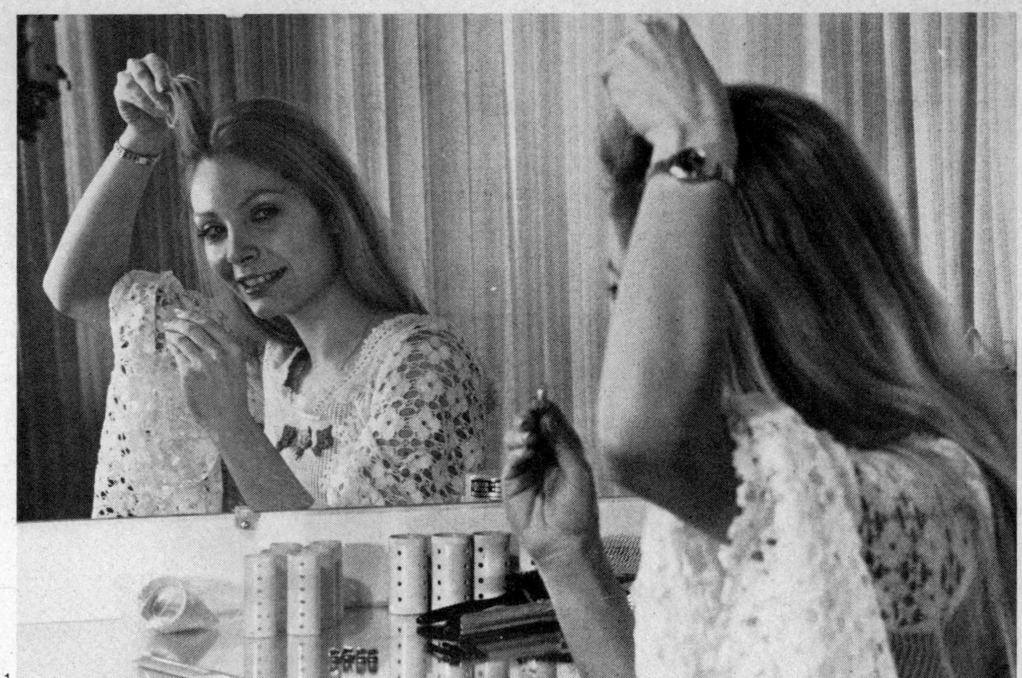

1 JON MARLOW

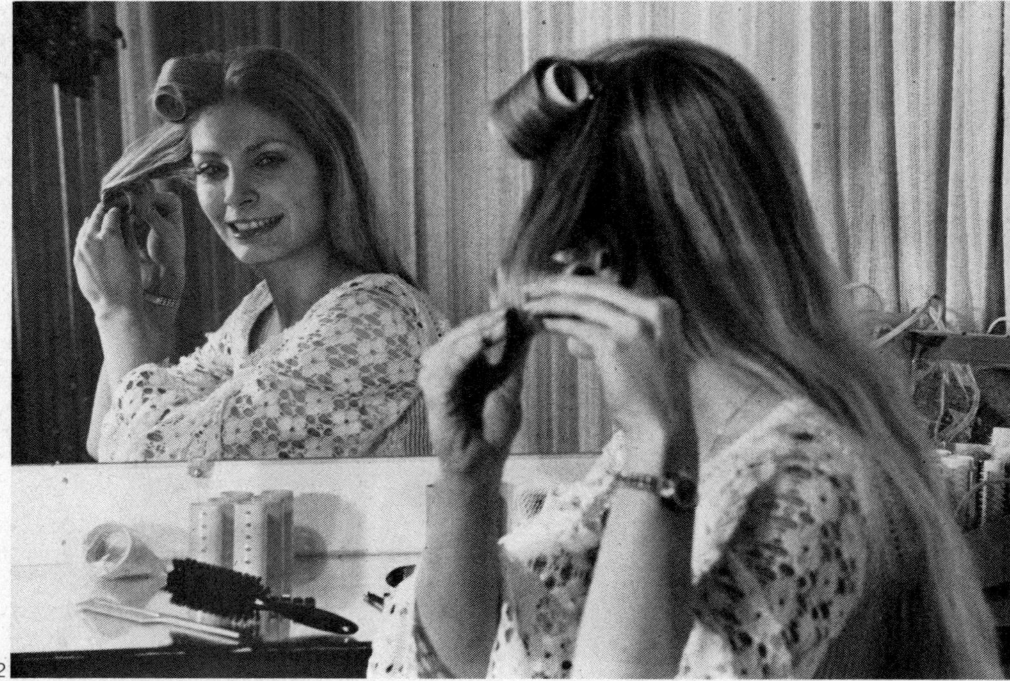

2

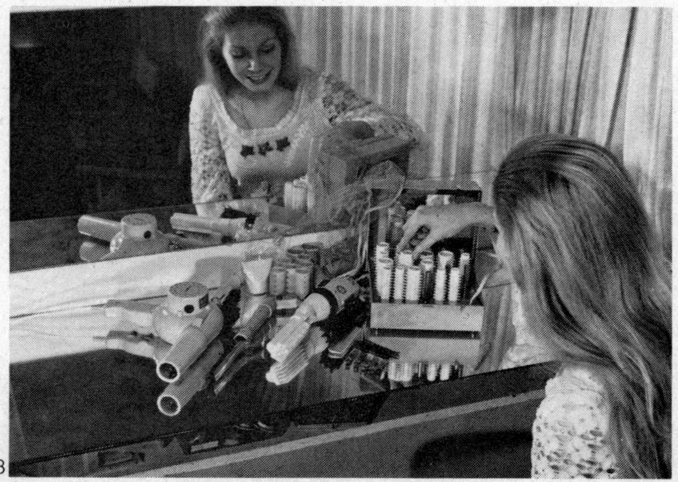

3

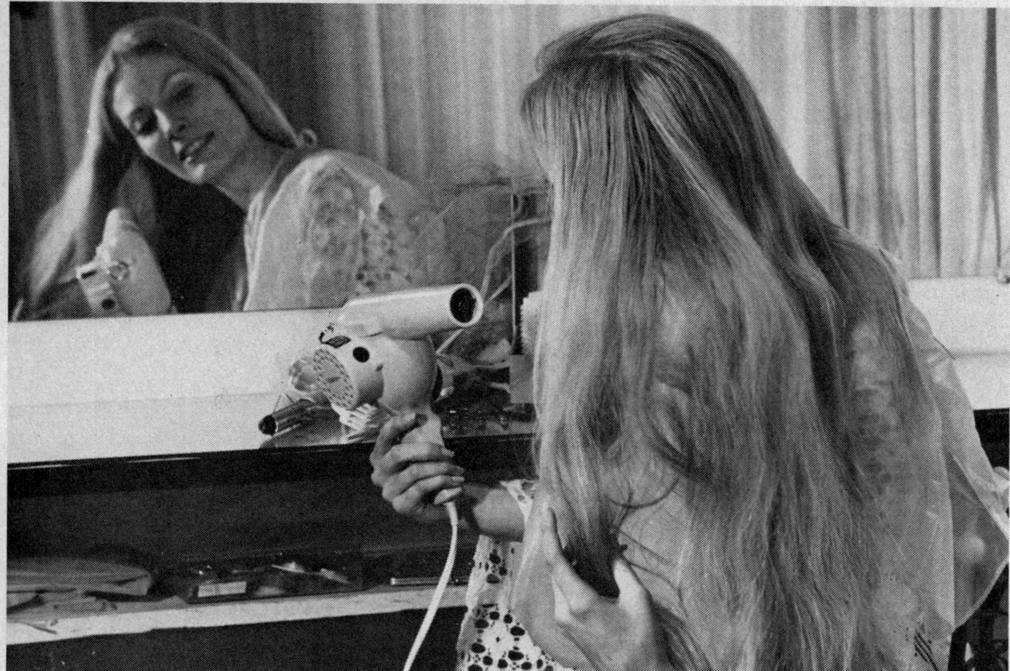

Large sections of teased hair will be layered, with the bottom layer brushed into position first, followed by sections on the middle layer, and finally the top.

Most back-combing or teasing at the sides of the hair involves back-combing the underside of each strand. If a "page-fluff" or a "flip" is desired, hair is brushed into flip position, teased on the underside and then smoothed from under the hair and over the hand. Unruly separations can be persuaded into place by tiny little back-combing strokes with the problem sections.

"Pageboy" or turned-under styles frequently need the extra body of a little back-combing of the underside of the hair, then brushed under the edge of the hand as it is held between hair and neck.

SPRAYING—A light hair spray is almost as necessary as film to a photographer working with a model. It should be used discriminately so the hair is disciplined without becoming stiff and unmovable. There are so many good sprays on the market, that it would serve no purpose to try to name them all—but a photographer should be equipped with a light and medium spray as well as a spray meant to enhance luster only such as Caryl Richards Happy Hair. □

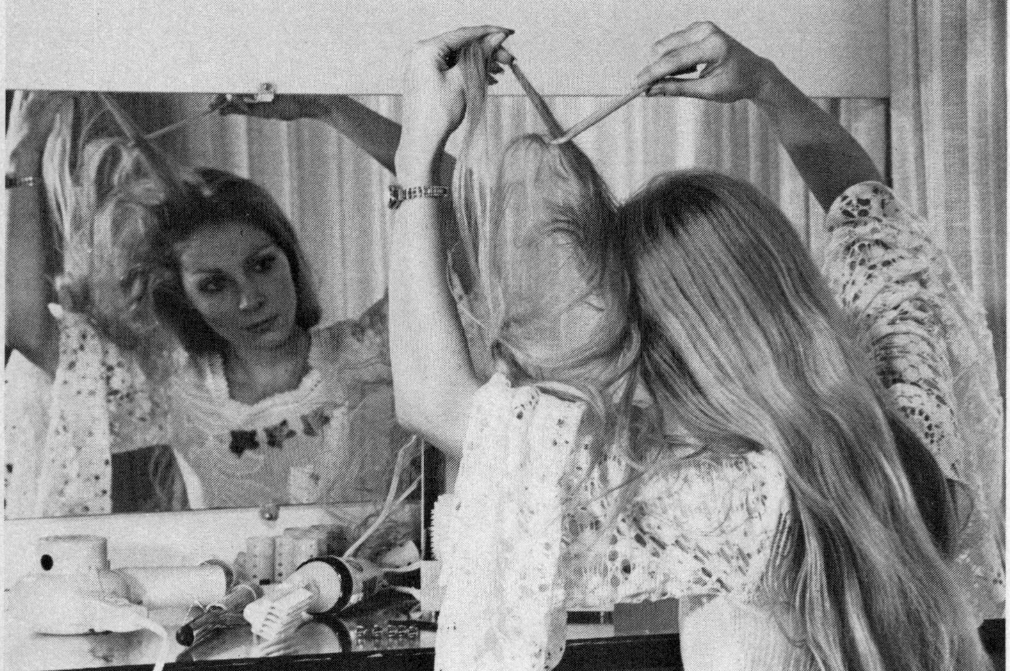

1. To set crown sections, hold strand straight up and away from scalp.
2. To set sides, strands should be pulled out and slightly upward before rolling.
3. Blower, brushes, combs and curlers should be on hand if photographer shoots models on a regular basis.
4. Blow dryer can be very handy.
5. Teasing hair involves grasping slim strands and holding firmly straight up from crown, and brushing or combing hair toward scalp, deliberately tangling it. Back-combing adds lift, body and fluffiness to hair.

the figure

It's a fairly well understood fact that a camera seems to add 10 or 12 pounds to a photographic subject and as a result, photo models, with the exception of matrons and characters, must be slimmer than average.

Aside from being slim, a model must be perfectly proportioned and have firm muscles. Even very slim models have found that when a camera freezes an action shot, the slightest amount of flab will show. In this sense, the demands of the still camera are greater than those of the motion picture camera. The viewer does not have time to catch as many of the details of the moving figure when the picture is in action.

Exercises and diet notwithstanding, most photographers find themselves frequently shooting models with less than perfect figures. Don't try to achieve the impossible. If her legs are short and fat, the photographer is wise to hide them. If she has a soft, too-rounded tummy and big hips, the string bikini is a poor choice.

But there are several tricks outside of actual concealment that can minimize figure flaws.

Legs look longer if the model stands on her toes or at least points the toe of the front leg (an obvious ploy, but nonetheless effective).

Heavy thighs will seem slimmer in a sitting pose with the model bending her knees. Thighs appear less visible if the model angles her knees slightly toward the camera.

Shapeless calves in a sitting pose can be made to seem rounder if the model angles her knees slightly toward the camera so the calf flesh falls toward the camera—use opposite technique for too-full calf.

Leg imperfections are less noticeable if legs are together—not necessarily straight, but with one leg bent slightly in front of the other.

Encourage the shorter, heavier model to experiment with straight line poses that involve a stretch rather than broken-line angles more suitable for the long, lanky girl.

Big hips will look larger when facing the camera straight on; teach the model to twist the hip (corresponding to the leg she's standing on) away from the camera.

Busty models need to emphasize—never hide—a small, stretched waistline to avoid looking plump in a full-length shot.

There are many more angles and tricks you and your model can discover with experimentation on her part, and your selective eye. But ideally, the model should be encourage to perfect her figure, rather than rely on camera tricks.

EXERCISES TO CORRECT FIGURE IMPERFECTIONS

SHOULDERS—Stand with legs slightly apart, arms out to the sides, shoulder height. Starting the movement from the shoulder sockets, move the arms and shoulders in large circles—eight forward circles and eight circles going backward. Now, make the circles going toward the ears and down again to shoulder height position.

BUST—Stand with legs slightly apart, hips tucked under. Grasp forearms in front of your body at shoulder height. Tighten grasp and jerk arms toward the elbows 50 to 75 times per night. Another method is to clasp hands behind you with heels of the hands touching. Keep the heels of the hands touching all the time as you straighten the elbows and lift arms up behind you as high as you can. Bounce arms upward around 10 times. Be sure to keep body straight.

WAIST—Stand with legs very far apart, grasping the elbows above the head. Bend from side to side around eight times. Or clasp hands above your head. Follow an imaginary circle and stretch hard as you twist from your torso—forward, side, back and side, in a large circular movement. Reverse directions.

TUMMY—Lie on your back, arms out to the side. Lift your legs slowly to the count of eight until toes are pointing straight up. Then, lower the legs until they are about 10 inches from the floor—spread wide apart, return together, then lower to the floor again. Do five times.

SWAY BACKS—Lie on the floor with the knees bent until heels are near the hips. Lift hips off the floor, and put waistline down first as you lower body back to the floor. Place your hands at the waistline and make sure that the waist is touching flat on the floor. Slowly straighten the legs while you maintain the flat waistline position.

HIPS—Lie on the floor with the knees bent up high near the chest, arms outstretched to the side at shoulder height. Keep the shoulders and arms on the floor as you twist from the waistline until knees are touching the floor at the left side. Now, straighten the legs, and keeping the heels about six inches from the floor, make a circle of the legs and bring them around to right side, bending the knees as you arrive in position. To tighten buttocks muscles, sit on the floor with the legs straight out in front of you. Keep your chest high, back straight. Walk on the hips across the room and back again. For the sides of the hips, lie on right side supporting the head on the right hand with the left hand on the floor in front of the body to balance you if necessary. Raise left leg to the side, then lower leg, 10 times. Repeat on the left side.

THIGHS—Stand on toes, take a step and bend the knees until you sit on the back heel, rise—take another step and repeat movement across the floor. (Knees should never touch the floor during excercise.) For the inside of the thighs sit on the floor with legs spread wide apart. Grasp ankles and bend forward. Try to touch forehead to the floor. Bounce forward eight times, then to the left knee eight times, to the right, then center again. To assure supple spine and backs of thighs assume standing position, bend over and grasp the ankles with the knees straight. Walk across the floor in this position.

CALVES AND ANKLES—Sit on the floor, back straight, point toes down—hold—then point toes up and backward toward the shins as far as they will go—hold position. Repeat. □

Ideally, the model should be slimmer than average, perfectly proportioned, with firm muscles.

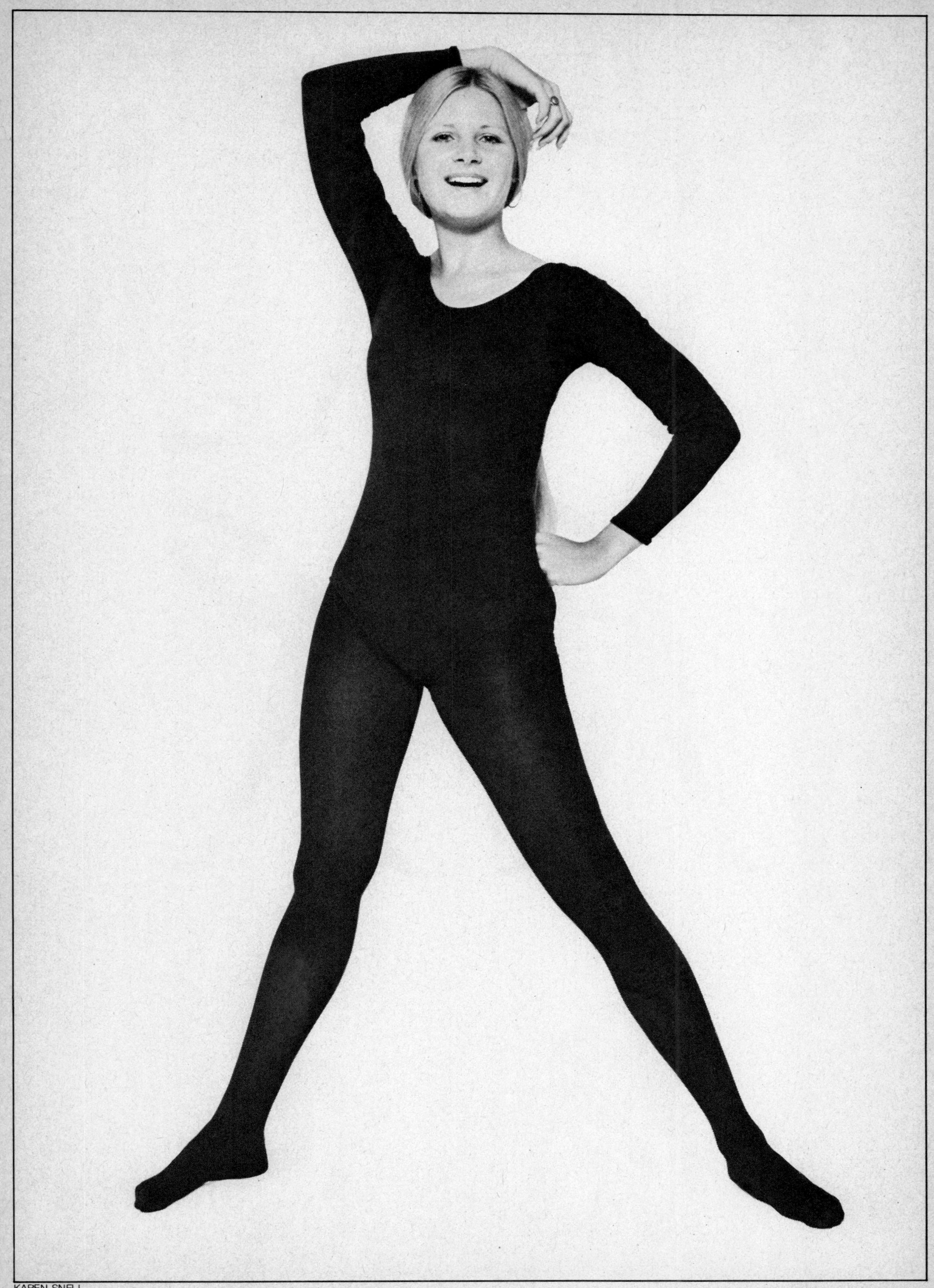

KAREN SNELL

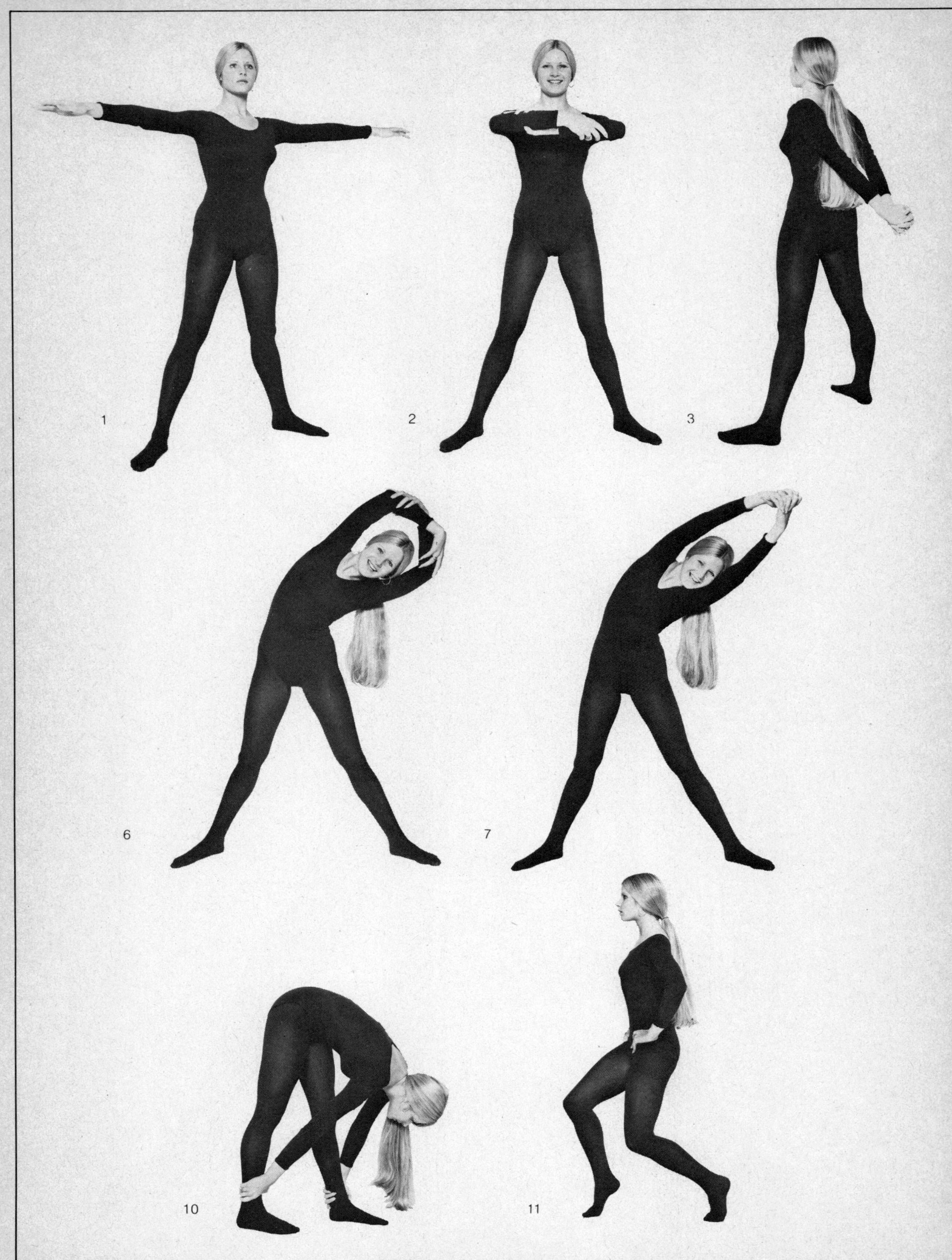

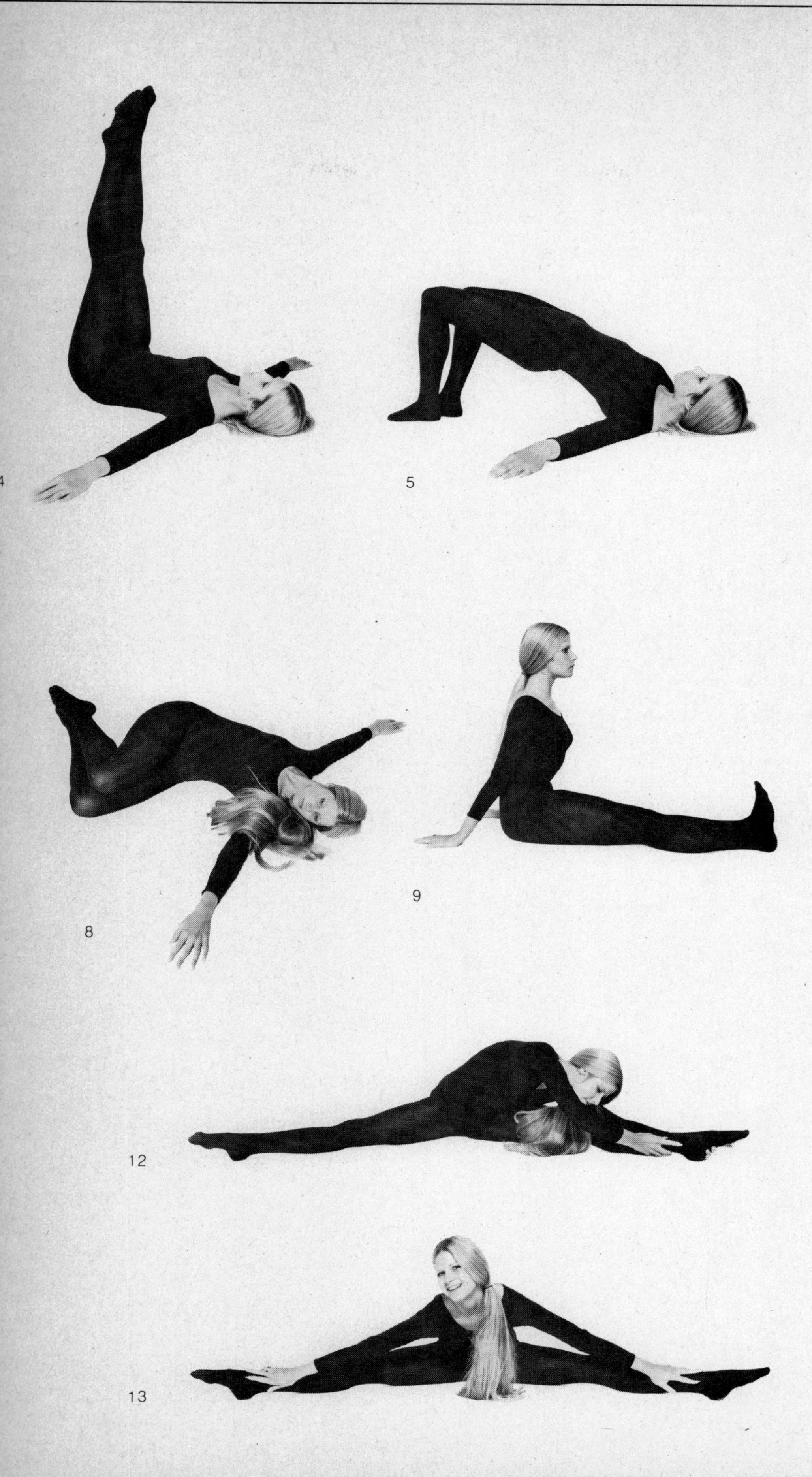

1. To shape up shoulders, start in this position and move arms and shoulders in large circles, first forward, then backward.

2. To firm up bust, assume this position, tighten grasp and jerk arms toward elbows 50 to 75 times per night.

3. Another bust exercise is to clasp hands behind you and straighten elbows and lift arms up as high as you can, keeping heels of hands touching.

4. For tummy, lie on back with arms out to sides. Lift legs slowly to count of eight until toes are pointing straight up, then lower legs until they are about 10 inches from floor, spread legs wide apart, return them together, then lower to floor. Do five times.

5. For sway backs, lie on floor with knees bent until heels are near hips. Lift hips off floor, and put waistline down first as you lower body back to floor. Slowly straighten legs while keeping waistline flat against floor.

6. For waist, assume this position and bend from side to side about eight times.

7. Another waist exercise is begun from this stance. Follow an imaginary circle and stretch hard as you twist torso forward, to side, back and side, then reverse directions.

8. For hips, lie on floor with knees bent up high near chest, arms outstretched to side at shoulder height. Keep shoulders and arms on floor as you twist from waistline until knees are touching floor at left side. Straighten legs and, keeping heels about six inches from floor, make circle of legs and bring them around to right side, bending knees as you arrive in that position (opposite of position illustrated).

9. To tighten buttocks muscles assume this position, and walk on hips across room and back.

10. To assure supple spine and backs of thighs, walk across floor in this position, keeping knees straight.

11. For thighs, stand on toes, take a step and bend knees until you sit on back heel, rise and take another step, and repeat movement across floor. Don't let knees touch floor.

12, 13. For inside of thighs, sit on floor with legs spread wide apart. Grasp ankles and bend forward, trying to touch floor with forehead. Bounce forward eight times, then to left knee eight times, to right knee and to center again.

potpourri

Except in fashion shots, in which the model is wearing the merchandise being featured in the photo, or in unique costume shots, a model is generally expected to provide her own wardrobe.

Professional models purchase their own wardrobe with their working needs in mind, avoiding black, too-busy prints or especially bulky lines. At least one bathing suit is protected from the water and saved just for pictures.

Your model should understand that she is responsible for the condition of her clothes. They must be absolutely spotless, perfectly pressed, in good condition and well accessorized. It is of utmost importance that the model consider her own type when selecting her personal/professional wardrobe. The junior model shouldn't buy siren-type clothes; the sophisticate shouldn't get too cute.

A photographer is well within his rights to expect a minimum wardrobe of current fashions consisting of: two or three bathing suits and at least two bathing suit cover-ups; a variety of colored tops, blouses and sweaters; at least two long dresses, preferably not of the bridesmaid variety of formals nor Empire cut which frequently photographs like a maternity dress; jeans (blue jeans, white ducks, faded denims, etc.); a couple of skirts (length of current fashions) and perhaps jackets and blazers to complement or match; pantsuits (dressier than jeans); a street-length cloth coat; a couple of hats—straw, knitted caps, felt brimmed, tennis, to name a few.

The photographer cannot reasonably expect, and should feel very lucky if his model can provide: special sports outfits (snow, ski, scuba wet-suits, English riding habit, etc.); costumes native to foreign countries; uniforms for nurses, stewardesses, waitresses, cheerleaders, etc.; bridal gowns; costumes and fashions common to another era. Nor can he expect the model to provide props or accessories such as skis, golf clubs, surfboards, ice or roller skates, cheerleading pompoms, etc.

It is the responsibility of the photographer to rent any unusual costume or prop such as these if his assignment or project requires them.

WARDROBE IN RELATION TO BACKGROUND

Every student of photography is aware of Avedon's famous surprises in contrasts—high fashion against backgrounds of wild animals, slums, trash, or half-finished constructions. As in all art, it takes a very sure hand to depart from the norm—rarely advisable for the novice photographer or model.

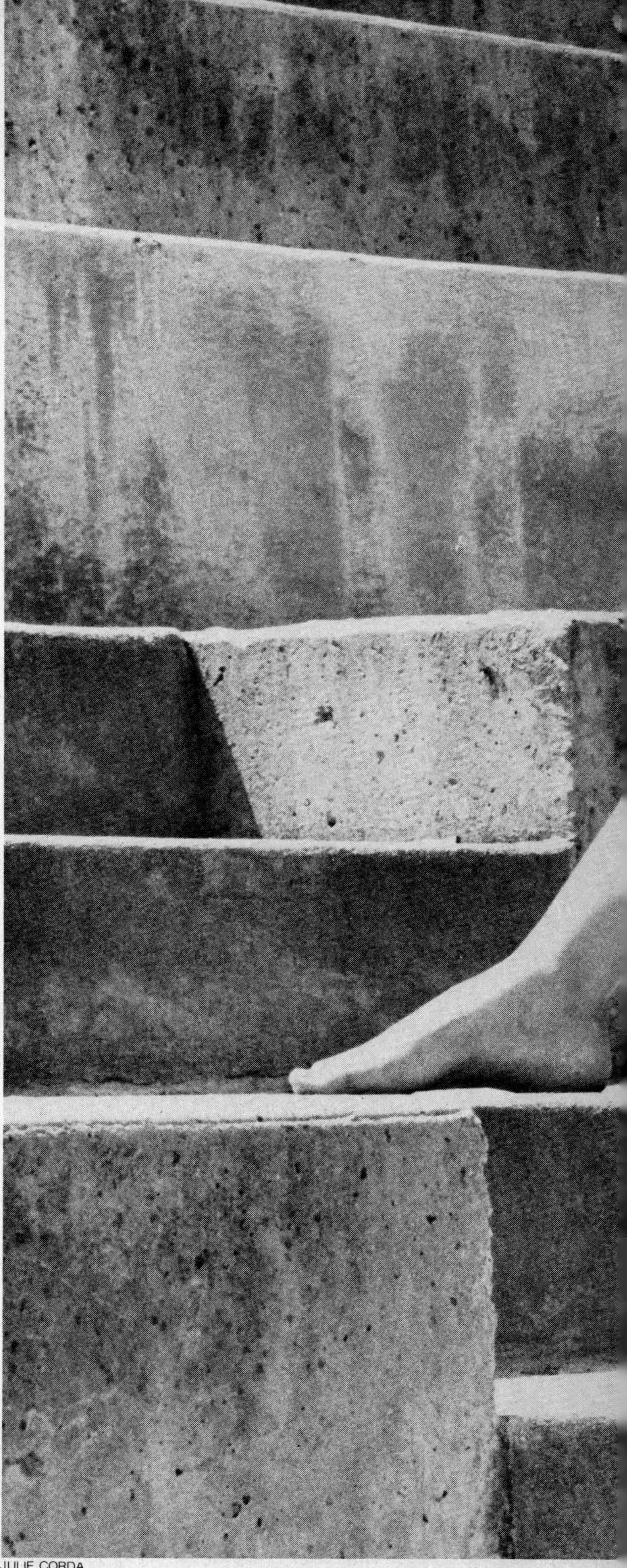

1. The model's clothes and the background are both part of the photo's environment, and special attention should be paid both.

JULIE CORDA

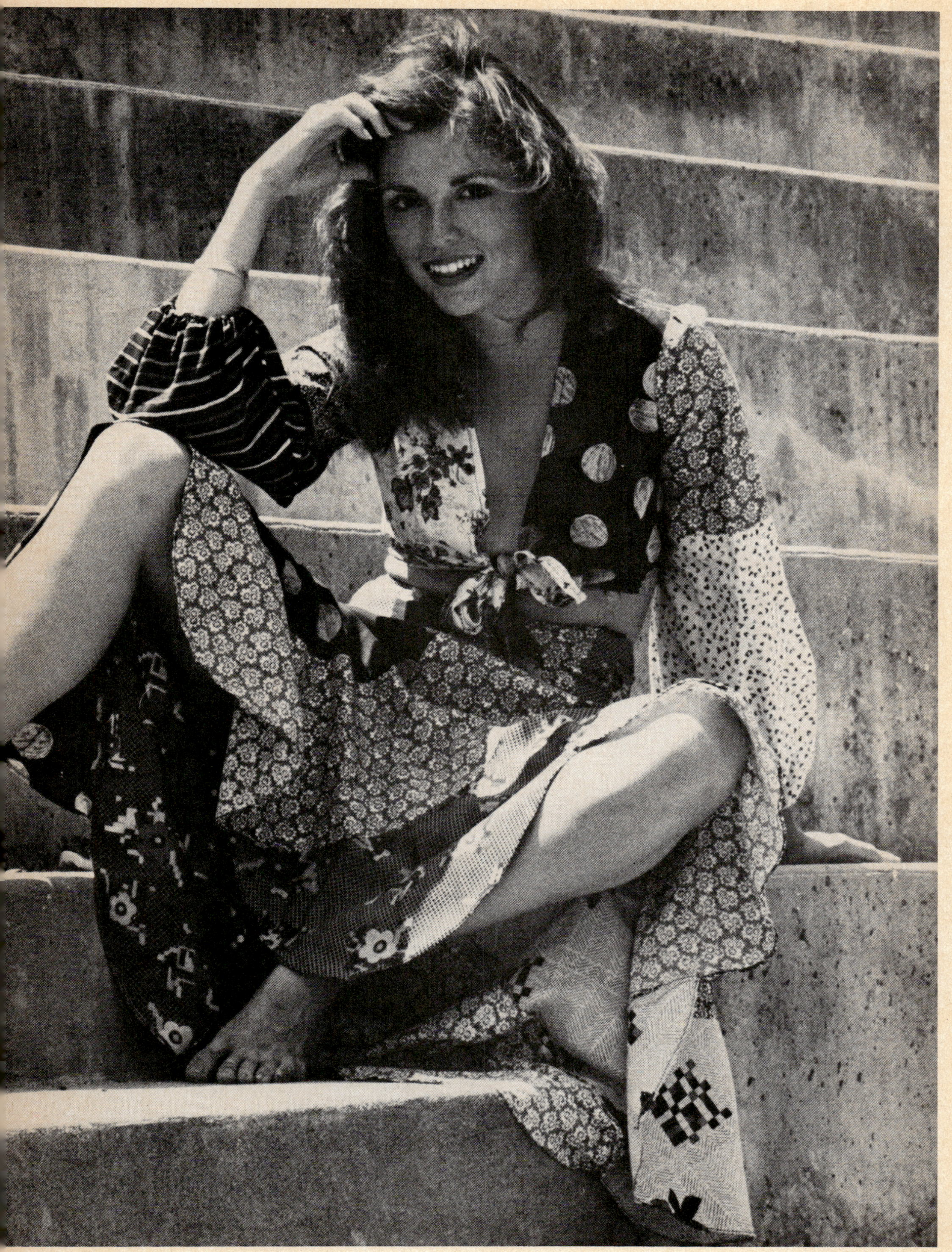

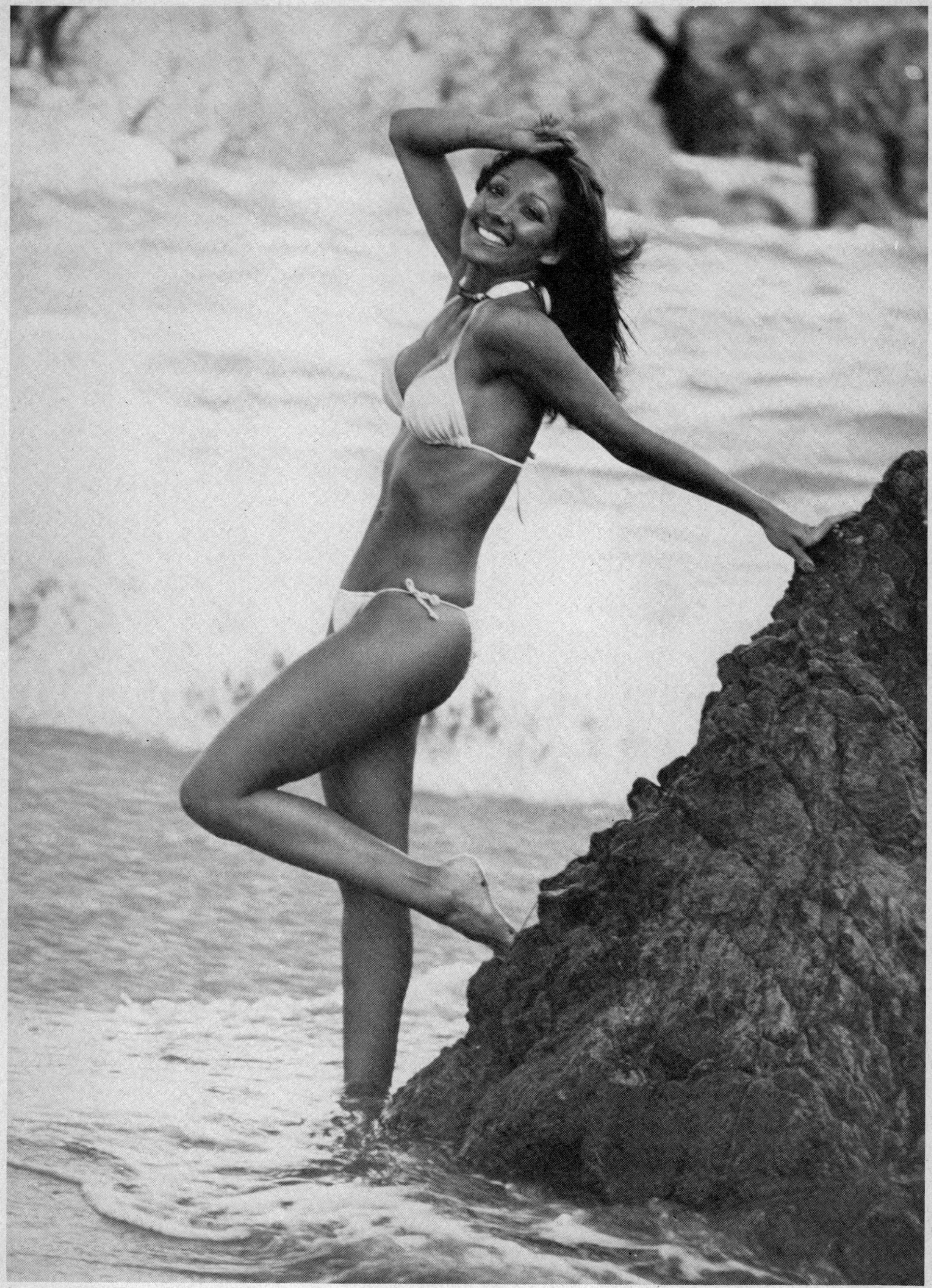

MINDI MILLER

VERTICAL	HORIZONTAL
Straight skirts	Very full skirts
Accordion-pleated skirts	Box-pleated skirts
Slash pockets	Large patch pockets
Stripes (vertical/thin)	Plaids
Solid colors	Contrasting colors, e.g., black skirt, white shirt
Matching, narrow belts	Wide and/or contrasting belts
Small caps (especially matching in tonal value)	Wide-brimmed hats and/or strongly contrasting with costume
Trim, such as buttons down the front	Horizontal trim, such as on a yoke, at waistline, or on pockets
Stockings matching garment	Stockings contrasting with garment
Shoes and/or tight boots same tonal value as garment	Shoes, boots contrasting with garment
Long sleeves, tight fitting	Large, full sleeves, raglan, puffed,
Dark tones	Light tones
Silk, jersey, chiffon, crepe, velvet, voile	Heavy wools, bulky satins, velveteens, startchy cottons, organdy, felt

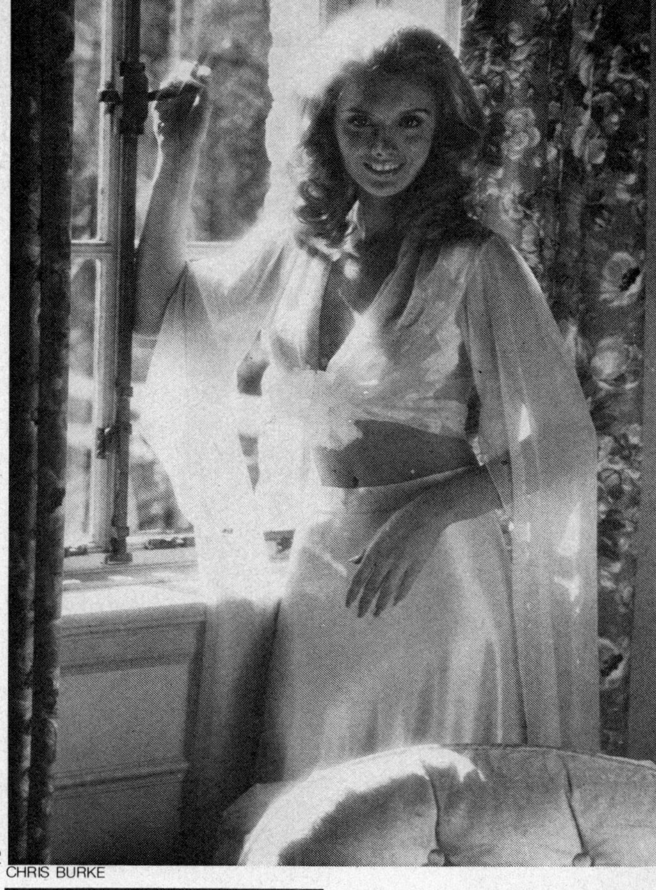

CHRIS BURKE

1. *Casual clothes fit into casual setting.*
2. *The clothes should match the mood of the photograph.*

Generally, the surest results can be achieved when the model's wardrobe and selected background are harmonious. With the above exception, clothes look best in the natural environment where they might conceivably be worn.

A model might be shot in a bathing suit in a wooded area, against mounds of sand, in or around a swimming pool or at a beach. Put her in a living room setting, on a residential front porch, or against a residential or business building, and you will most likely be assured of a garish or incongruous effect.

Consider your locations carefully with regard to the fashions your model will be wearing. Today's trend seems to be moving more and more into the candid, slice-of-life situational shot. Ideally, your photo should tell a story. Don't try to get too complicated—keep the situation and background simple. But do consider the special impact that relevancy in fashion and background can have.

LINES, TONAL VALUES, AND FABRICS

It is also important for the photographer to be aware of impressions and optical illusions created by lines, tone values of colors (or colors in color photography) and bulk in fabrics. Vertical lines and soft, clinging fabrics generally make the model appear taller and slimmer. Horizontal lines and bulky fabrics add width to the model and make her appear somewhat shorter. Check the examples on the horizontal/vertical line chart to help you and your models become aware of these effects.

THE MODEL'S COMPENSATION

A photographer should make it an unfailing rule to compensate a model for working for him. Professional models have definite rates established by their modeling agencies and, if a professional model is being used for a commercial assignment, she will expect her regular rates. Modeling rates vary throughout the country, and according to the model. In large cities, where models are used regularly (such as New York, Chicago, Los Angeles), rates vary from $45 an hour to $75 an hour—with a few superstars in New York demanding and getting more. The daily rate is five times that of the model's hourly rate ($250 for a $50-an-hour model, $300 for a $60-an-hour model). Exceptional New York models will not take a daily rate. If the job is a "catalogue" assignment, the rate is $5 an hour less than a model's usual fee.

Contracts involving exclusivity of a model's appearance on any competing product involve special compensation depending upon the area in which a model is working and the likelihood of her losing employment due to the exclusivity arrangement.

Most agencies bill extra for traveling time outside of the city in which the model is employed—usually half pay. Sometimes travel fees are waived—it really depends upon the job, how many days the model will be working, among other factors.

Outdoor location assignments are frequently booked on a *weather-permitting* basis, varying upon the agency and the size of the modeling business in the particular location. Many agencies will waive any charge if the weather does not permit shooting while some charge half fee. In either case, the concerned parties must be notified well in advance of the cancellation—certainly not after the model has arrived at the location. There are commercial jobs, of course, for which the photographer will be paid and this naturally means the model will be paid also, but there are some shooting situations in which neither the photographer nor the model will profit financially. Instead they are shooting for a mutual need to build up their portfolios, artistic experimentation, or even just for fun. In this event, the model should get the same thing for her time that the photographer is getting—pictures.

It's important to make the arrangements specific and be certain they are agreed upon in advance. The very minimum compensation a model is entitled to is one 11x14 or two 8x10 prints for each proof sheet or one print for every 16 to 20 shots taken.

At any rate, the model should receive at least three to six pictures for an afternoon's shooting—any less, and it's not worth her time. On the other hand, a photographer is unwise indeed to tell a model she may have ''whatever she likes'' after she sees the proofs—she may expect and ask for much more than her time was worth.

CONCLUSION

Introducing someone to the modeling experience or, perhaps, even a full-blown career can carry with it inherent responsibilities— responsibilities that seem to have eluded the media of today.

The media, and all those in its periphery, including photographers, clients and modeling agencies, have conceived and given birth to the *media-monster*—or *media-princess,* if you will. Because of the media's ever-increasing influence on all of us, the *monster* has become an established value in our lives—much to the chagrin of roughly 99.9 percent of the remaining women in the extremely impressionable populace of this country. This false ideal has become so entrenched in the minds of the consumer that she (the monster-princess) is now one of the most powerful sales tools, ever.

Let's take a look at her for a moment, from a totally objective point of view, and try to understand just what it is that makes her so irresistible to the American public. She falls somewhere between 5-feet-6 and 5-feet-9, is around 16 to 25 years old, is small-boned and slim, has perfectly straight teeth, a beautiful, flawless complexion, and has a 70 percent chance of being a blue-eyed blond. If a model just happens to fall within these narrow descriptive confines, she can probably realize a lucrative, exciting and ego-satisfying career.

But this is where the tragedy of it all comes in—this concept, especially as prevalent as it has become, is a poor criterion indeed by which to judge a lady's worth. The photographer and the model must recognize the invalidity of this premise that bone structure is somehow related to the model's self-esteem and value of herself—but is indeed simply a fortunate accident.

If the plastic prettiness of our princess were all that was required, we then could, of course, simply utilize a papier-mache mannequin in photographic presentations— much less expensively, too, we might add.

But let's not forget the human element—the thought, mood and energy that brings a model-oriented photograph to life. The model can offer a wide, deep range of rich personality while the photographer, in turn, exercises discrimination and selectivity when he chooses that aspect of her individuality he wants to present to the viewer.

The good photographer will help his model by his attitude toward her to look beyond her mask of beauty and regard her effort as a creative experience— emphasizing this element of her work can offer her the opportunity of full expression. The photographer, then, will be able to share creative moments with his model that will bring a new and special dimension to his life and labor. □